GO
ONE
MORE

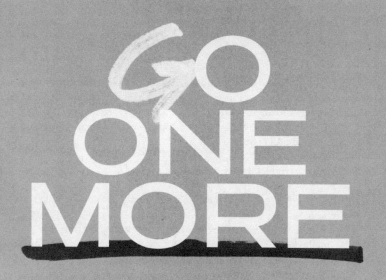

GO
ONE
MORE

FIND THE CLARITY TO
MAKE INTENTIONAL,
LIFE-CHANGING
CHOICES

NICK BARE

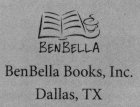

BenBella Books, Inc.
Dallas, TX

The events, locations and conversations in this book, while true, are recreated from the author's memory. However, the essence of the story, and the feelings and emotions evoked are intended to be accurate representations. In certain instances, names, persons, organizations, and places have been changed to protect an individual's privacy.

Go One More copyright © 2025 by Nick Bare

BenBella Books, Inc.
8080 N. Central Expressway
Suite 1700
Dallas, TX 75206
benbellabooks.com
Send feedback to feedback@benbellabooks.com

BenBella is a federally registered trademark.

Printed in the United States of America
10 9 8 7 6 5 4 3 2 1

Library of Congress Control Number: 2024057549
ISBN 9781637746219 (hardcover)
ISBN 9781637746226 (electronic)

Editing by Victoria Carmody
Copyediting by Lyric Dodson
Proofreading by Ashley Casteel and Jenny Bridges
Text design and composition by Jordan Koluch
Cover design by Ethan Davis
Printed by Sheridan MI

This book is dedicated to my children.

We have a responsibility to build a life filled with purpose and impact. I encourage you to work hard and chase your wildest ambitions. But in that process, don't forget to live, play, and be present with the people you love.

Contents

The only constant we can expect is change. It will happen whether we fight it or invite it. The summation of our life's choices will determine the success we achieve and the fulfillment we experience from those decisions. The question differs from how we react to change to how prepared we are to adapt and evolve. We need clarity to make intentional, life-changing choices and create a legacy that reaches our most significant potential.

Introduction

THE ORIGIN STORY

*W*hy keep going?

I asked myself this question nine miles into an eighteen-mile training run for my first marathon in 2018. I was in downtown Austin on a cold and damp day, running the loop around Lady Bird Lake, also known as Town Lake by the local Austinites. As I approached mile ten, my legs began to ache and feel heavy. I felt tired, and I didn't feel like running. Voices in my head kept giving me reasons to stop.

You're not a runner. You're too big to be a runner.

You don't know anything about running. What are you even doing out here?

Didn't you run enough in the military? You've got more important things going on in your life now. Get back to work.

This is what running does. Mile after mile, your body and your will begin to break down and fatigue. Eventually, you'll be hurting, and every part of you will scream for you to slow down and stop. Your body will beg you, sending your mind every signal it can to tell you it's tired and needs rest. The mind naturally favors the path of least resistance; however, it also drives your body to keep pushing through those challenges.

Some of life's greatest rewards are on the other side of that resistance.

On this day, I stopped and started walking back to the house that I was renting after those first ten miles. Nobody was there to watch. Nobody was going to know that I chose to avoid the resistance. But with each step I took, different thoughts flooded my mind. I began to argue with myself. Here I was, running a successful business that just crossed the seven-figure revenue mark, building a brand for my company and myself, and preparing to get married. Yet I was quitting.

If I quit on this run now, what will that say about my character? What else in my life will I give up on?

I turned around and forced myself to go back and finish that run. By the time I crossed the eighteen-mile mark, I didn't pat myself on the back.

I kept going.

I ran one more mile. One more than I was originally planning.

When I got back home, I took my hat off and wrote two simple words on the bill: one more.

I wrote them for myself—as a reminder for the next time and the time after that. Then for fun, I took a photo of it and posted it on social media to share my story. To my surprise, the post blew up, with all these people writing "one more" on the bill of their hats. I realized this phrase and mindset struck a nerve in people. I modified it to make it something more profound:

Go One More.

Three words. Three simple words that I got tattooed on my arm as a daily reminder that my ability, my bandwidth, and my tank always have a little bit left inside them. I can always push a little further even when it's tough. The tattoo is a constant reminder that we all have more ability than we think. Hundreds, if not thousands, of other people were so moved by this message that they got these three words tattooed on their bodies as well.

Go One More is about more than the extra miles. It's about more than an extra rep. It's about more than an extra day's work. It is the compounding consistency of putting in the extra effort every single day. This mantra suddenly changed the trajectory of my work, providing me with the direction I needed to fulfill my life's mission and a determination to help many others do so as well. But this is just the beginning.

This book isn't just about that mantra. It's about what comes next.

I came up with Go One More when I came to the realization that I was making a mistake by deciding to quit my training run. I realized my decision was influenced by weakness, and I decided to reject that weakness and pursue greatness. Ultimately, by choosing to Go One More, I was striving for an outcome, but I didn't have the perspective or the depth of thought to realize that at the time. I just thought of Go One More as an action. I thought that just doing more of anything would lead me to overwhelming success. That outcome was much greater than a short-term gain. It was a habit that would be forged through the consistent choice of Go One More in everything I did from that point on.

I'm going to run one more mile, and if I run one more mile or I do one more thing, that will compound over time. And if I keep doing that, that compounding consistency builds and builds and builds.

That is true for certain things as long as you're intentional and strategic with what you are working on. But I've discovered that just the action of "Going" One More does not facilitate the outcome that you might be trying to achieve.

I've come across so many people—and I've done this myself on a lot of projects, challenges, and pursuits—who think that just by doing the work, they will be rewarded with the outcome. It doesn't necessarily matter what the work is. Sometimes, we think that just doing *more* of something or working harder on anything will get us to our goal, but just because you're working harder doesn't mean you deserve the outcome. It doesn't mean you've *earned* it. The work we put in needs to be strategic, intentional, and very thoughtful to have the outcome we want and desire.

Go One More is not just an action. It's an outcome.

You may hear Go One More and think of it as a verb, but it's more than that. Go One More is a results-driven mindset. By applying this mindset to everything you do, you will unlock opportunities and growth in life that will set you up for success years from now. It's more than doing more. It's doing more of the right things, at the right time, for the right reasons.

The Mission

The reason I'm writing this book is to share how the meaning and message of Go One More has evolved for me personally. As my children grow up, they can reference these lessons and stories to create a life filled with success and impact that builds off a foundation of personal values. I've learned that, in order to apply and experience Go One More in your life, you need clarity. Clarity on what you are working on, why you are working on it, and how you are working to achieve that thing. Without the what, why, and how, you are just doing stuff. And through doing, you are hoping and wishing that just by doing more of something, it will pay off. But that's not necessarily how it works. Go One More is the outcome, not necessarily just the action. It's the intention behind the what, why, and how.

Why do I document and share my life? I don't have all the answers. I'm not a guru. I'm not always the smartest person in any room I walk into. But I do have lots of courage. I take action on things I'm curious about, and in that process, I succeed at some and fail at others. I learn a lot through those lessons. I'm constantly reading, learning, teaching, sharing, leading, and following. I gain a lot from all of it, and I get a lot of fulfillment from sharing it. I like seeing the positive impact it makes on others. When something works for me, I want everyone to know so they can reap the benefits, too. That's what this book is. It's not a book of answers, but it is a collection of personal learnings that I feel obligated to share.

I really admire wisdom. It's one reason I love to interview people on my podcast and why I'm constantly reading. I don't think you acquire wisdom just through age, but rather through time and experience. These stories and lessons are a collection of the wisdom I've gained and experienced. My hope is that it will help people in the different chapters of their lives. One of my favorite podcasts is called *Founders* by David Senra. He shares the lives, stories, and work ethics of the world's most successful entrepreneurs, athletes, and leaders. His show description quotes Marc Andreessen by saying, "There is so much more to learn from the past than we often realize. You could productively spend your time reading experiences of great people who have come before and you learn every time."

This isn't a how-to book. I don't like telling people how to live their lives. But my hope is that it will create and spark clarity and perspective. With that, people can make their own decisions about how to live the life that allows them to achieve the outcome of going one more. My ultimate goal is to get you to think about the choices you make on a daily basis that guide the trajectory of your life. This book is a guide to help you avoid making the mistakes I've made. Every piece of advice I share I learned because I messed up along the way—not prioritizing my family, being selfish, losing track of my meaningful mission, and feeling completely lost when it looks like I've had it all figured out from the outsider's perspective.

By setting the conditions and building a foundation for personal success, you have the capacity to impact others. These chapters and stories are about how I'm learning to live a more intentional life and how clarity allows me to help others do the same. I not only want you to find success and clarity and experience the power of Go One More, but to also leave a legacy that carries on for generations to follow.

Chapter One

PURSUE INTENTIONALITY

"The man who loves walking will walk further than the man who loves the destination."

—Lao Tzu

What truth am I going to unlock today?

The question intrigued me. It was the reason I ventured to Pineland Farms, Maine, in
September of 2023 to do a backyard ultramarathon called
Last Man Standing. This wasn't an ordinary ultra. This was
a 4.2-mile loop that restarted every hour, on the hour, until
only one person was left. Runners couldn't start early or late.
With each loop, the distance and the duration increased, and
so did the damage to your body. There would only be one
winner. Everyone else would be considered a DNF.

Did not finish.

I had finished two ultramarathons before I entered Last Man Standing: the Leadville Trail 100, an out-and-back race across the Rocky Mountains of Colorado, and the Rocky Raccoon, a one-hundred-mile trail run that consists of five twenty-mile loops through the woods of east Texas. This time, I was looking for something new and different. I knew how to plan, strategize, and complete a one-hundred-mile race, but an ultramarathon that simply told you to run as far as you possibly could while restricting how far you could go every hour? This approach was new, and there were so many unknowns to it. It presented an opportunity to unlock a unique perspective. That was exactly why I signed up for it.

Fitness has always been a large part of my identity. It has been more than a passion; it's my work. When I entered the Last Man Standing, I was at a point in my life when my relationship with fitness had evolved. My business and family had grown, my priorities had shifted, and as a result, my ambitious physical challenges had to provide me with more than just an extra notch on the belt. There had to be an "unlock." I'm not someone who signs up for these events to collect bibs or medals, and I never have been, because the meaning behind the process is much deeper than that to me. It's never been about something to hang my hat on, but to learn from. I've proved that I can commit to a goal, be hyper-focused through the weeks and months leading up to it, and show up prepared to execute. For years, I have been running marathons, ultras, and triathlons. I've pushed my body to the ultimate extremes, trained for hours a day, and became surprisingly efficient at burning the candle at both ends—something I don't actively promote but needed to do in the early stages of my career. In my opinion, setting out to accomplish something in order to prove others wrong is a dead end. It's a pursuit to achieve external validation, and that approach no longer resonated with me.

Going into Last Man Standing, I didn't have this burning desire to win the race. The concept of running one hundred miles didn't intimidate me since I had covered that distance in ultras before. For this race, I was hoping to unlock something that I had been working on for some time. I wanted to know how Go One More had evolved for me. I had felt the shift but couldn't articulate it. It was on the tip of my tongue, but putting it into words felt impossible. The physical, mental, and emotional suffering that we are able to experience through something challenging provides us with the ability to unlock new compartments of our minds, but we have to set the conditions for it to happen. My hope was that an event like Last Man Standing could facilitate the breakthrough I needed.

When I lined up with the other runners at the start of the race, I couldn't help but think about how different things were from three years ago at the Austin Marathon. Back then, I ran to prove myself wrong—to prove other people wrong. But this race—and this year—was all about proving myself right.

Prove Yourself Right

Motivation. We all need it. Or maybe I should say we all *want* it. Many people seek an external motivating force to flood their brains with a strong release of dopamine, a neurotransmitter and hormone that affects our emotions, behavior, and movement and helps us feel pleasure as part of the brain's reward system. But what if that force could be internally created instead? What if your superpower really comes from being internally motivated?

When I decided to start Bare Performance Nutrition (BPN), I told my dad I was going to make one million dollars that year. I'll never forget his response.

"Nick, if it were that easy, everyone would do it."

That was all the fuel I needed. I set out to prove him wrong, an external motivation born through a desire to gain praise and approval from my father. But he was right: it wasn't easy. We generated about $20,000 in revenue that first year, and it took five long and grueling years before BPN finally reached the seven-figure mark.

I'm a big fan of self-motivation and personal drive, but I've discovered a ground-breaking concept in the last few years. We need to flip the script that often drives us. Instead of trying to prove ourselves and others wrong, we need to prove ourselves right. Part of me has always had this mindset. I've never been someone who thought deep down, *I'm going to prove him wrong*, or, *I'm going to show them*. That was never the reason I worked so hard and wanted to accomplish my big dreams and aspirations. I longed for those dreams and aspirations. I believed in them and was fully passionate about them. Yet, for many years, there was always this voice in the back of my head that reminded me of my doubters. A voice that replayed their skepticism.

You can't do that, Nick. You're not going to succeed.

There have been times I've tried to use that as fuel. Like when one of my bosses doubted me during my transition out of the Army. He wanted me to fail and told me I would regret leaving the military because my business wasn't going to work. Then, in 2019, I announced on social media that I was going to train for the 2020 Austin Marathon and run it in under three hours. My best marathon before this was three hours and fifty-seven minutes. Ambitious, right? The amount of doubt that rolled in from personal messages and across online forums was profound. While this doubt provided me with a trace amount of fuel, it also started to instill doubt in me, which is incredibly dangerous. The truth is, doubt is only dangerous when you start doubting yourself. I ran that marathon in three hours and twenty-four minutes—a significant miss. The doubters loved every one of those twenty-four minutes over my goal time.

So then I refined my plan, shifted my mindset, trained for another year, and ran a marathon in two hours, fifty-six minutes, and twenty-seven seconds. Goal accomplished. What changed? In that last year of training, I set out to prove *to myself* that I could do it. I did it for me and no one else, especially not for the people who said I couldn't.

At different stages of my life, I've set out to achieve a goal for the sole purpose of competing with someone or something else. Some people are able to use that as their only source of fuel and motivation, but I've never been able to resonate with that mentality. I'm not here to tell you that one way is better than the other, but I am here to share with you what has worked for me. When I've tried to use external validation, "proving others wrong" or "having a chip on my shoulder" as motivation to succeed, it never felt right. It was never fulfilling, and it came from a place of insecurity—not strength or confidence. Working from a place of insecurity in this way only guided me toward emotional decisions instead of rational ones. There is nothing fulfilling to me about accomplishments that result in a *Ha, I got you!* Accomplishments should be confidence boosters. They should be stepping stones that generate momentum for the next big, ambitious goal.

Sometimes, you can make the mistake of trying to prove *yourself* wrong, like I did with my sub-three-hour marathon attempt in 2020. I didn't believe in myself so much, and I wrote "You fucking can't" on my arm in bold, black Sharpie, right under my Go One More tattoo. I knew the marathon was going to be very challenging and that finishing in under three hours would be tough. I wanted to be able to look down at my arm and tell myself, *Nick, you can't do this. No one believes in you. You gotta prove yourself and all those other doubters wrong.*

So guess what happened? The exact thing I had scrawled on my arm happened.

This was the wrong approach to take because it was built on the fact that I didn't believe in myself, that I didn't believe in what I was trying to do.

It was self-sabotage, an attempt to accomplish my goal from a place of insecurity rather than confidence.

So, why not try to prove yourself right instead? This approach indicates that you believe in your potential and the outcome. You believe in the result. Of course, you have to be committed and disciplined to see the process through, but it's an internally driven desire. And it's achievable. Anything is achievable. That's the way I think about it. Don't try to prove anybody else wrong. Don't even try to prove yourself wrong. Be intentional about proving yourself right.

At the start of 2023, I challenged the BPN community to prove themselves right by choosing something new and hard to be a part of. Commitment was the first step, enduring the process was the second, and executing on the goal was the third. Each step is equally important and necessary to experience growth and success in all aspects of life.

Of course, I took part in the challenge as well and decided to participate in three events. First, I entered a bodybuilding show, which was something very different than my last couple years of training had prepared me for. Different meant discomfort in the process, and I needed that. The second was Last Man Standing, and the third was finishing a marathon in under two hours and forty-five minutes. The process that was required by these three separate goals was very unique, but the foundation of success remained the same: commit, endure, and execute. During my time in the military, we followed an eight-step training model. It was tried, tested, and true. This three-step process produced similar results for my life post-military.

In order to prove yourself right, you need to stop trying to prove others wrong. And to do that, you need to be, what I call, *self-powered*.

Be Self-Powered

As I said, the times I tried to use proving others wrong as motivation never worked out for me. People who are constantly trying to prove others wrong are powered by their criticism, pessimism, negativity, and disbelief. But when you're self-powered, you are driven by an internal belief and a true unique confidence in yourself. It is the most powerful and potent fuel source in the world. If you can figure out a way to bottle that up and sell it, you will be richer than those who own the oil fields and distribute it across the world.

Being self-powered is where drive and discipline meet confidence. In one of my favorite books, *Winning* by Tim Grover, he talks about the importance of stacking wins throughout a lifetime. Your first win is difficult but also extremely rewarding. This could be graduating from college, your first job promotion, starting a business, or accomplishing another goal, milestone, or significant life event. The definition of a win is broad and specific to you. That first win comes with a new level of confidence that you didn't have before, and each additional win you achieve after that first one is harder, but builds more and more confidence. After practicing this for years, you become a self-powered machine that thrives under pressure with a remarkable amount of confidence in your ability to do anything you set your mind and body to. As you stack these wins, you can't ignore the fact that they are accompanied by just as many, if not more, losses. These losses are necessary, so don't be afraid to fail forward because it is still momentum, and momentum is potential.

Ever since I can remember, I've been self-powered. It wasn't always the strongest force within me, but it has become stronger over the years. I think some of those traits were built into my DNA, things I inherited and learned from both sides of my family, things that have shaped who I am.

My dad's family were dairy farmers. He and his brother grew up working hard on their father's farm. It wasn't a very affectionate family, but I think that's just the nature of the business. My grandpa was often stressed out from keeping track of the weather conditions, the crop yield, and how much money they were making on milk and the cows. A small farming operation is a hard business and a hard life. Every morning at 4 AM, you're milking cows, and every night before going to bed, you're milking cows again. This way of life is focused around work. Work is survival, and there are no off days or vacations. Naturally, there is an emotionless quality about it, where you make objective decisions based on what has to be done and not necessarily what you want to do.

My mom's side of the family was different. Many of them were in the military and worked in blue-collar jobs. They were very warm, loving, and empathetic. Anytime my grandmother saw you, she'd pull you in, kiss you all over, and embrace you. She sometimes started crying simply because she was so excited to see you. Mom grew up in a small home with a one-acre garden in the backyard. Every Sunday after church, we went to their house for homemade burgers and French fries. The hand-picked lettuce, tomatoes, and onions all came from my grandpa's garden, and so did the corn on the cob. Meals together would be full of laughter and conversation.

Over the years, I've come to appreciate the dynamics of both families because I've learned and acquired characteristics and traits from both sides. There are times when I can be very stoic and very objective. Sometimes I can be cold and remove emotion from my decision-making. I'm able to detach myself from a situation and look at it from an unbiased, third-party view. I learned that from my dad's side of the family, the dairy farmers. But I also can be warm, empathetic, loving, caring, and understanding—all the things my mom's side of the family embodied. I've realized that I can move from the emotional to the logical like the flip of a switch. It feels seamless. While both sides of my family were very different, they were both self-powered. They were driven, ambitious, and hard-working people who wanted to build a better life for themselves and the people around them. This way of life never had to be discussed because it was simply what they practiced daily and instilled in me. My family has been instrumental to my success, leadership, and determination.

I don't share this information to say that you must come from a self-powered lineage to inherit these skills and characteristics. I share my experience to show that being self-powered is a value that is reinforced by consistency and practice. It doesn't matter if you grew up working on a farm, served in the military, or operated as a C-suite executive for a Fortune 500 company. Being self-powered is a responsibility we each have the ability to embrace, live out, and pass on to the generations that come after us.

I see being self-powered as this internal drive of motivation and discipline. You are not trying to compete against someone else or prove anyone else wrong. You aren't trying to fake it, either. A true internal vision and mission drives you. This feeling is an intuition that forms in the gut. Sometimes you can't explain the what, why, or how, but it's there.

When you are self-powered, you are completely in control. You remove the impulse to please others, and you maximize execution. I can say that I'm self-powered, and you can, too. It is a choice that requires intentionality, discipline, and ruthless consistency. This isn't a quality that you are either born with or without. It is a skill that can be practiced and forged through repetition. If there is something you want to turn into a habit, you just have to apply frequency of repetition to it on a consistent basis. Do that long enough and that action will eventually become habitual—for better or worse.

Imagine being completely reliant on a fuel source to get through a day's work and life's mission. Like someone struggling with addiction requires their daily dose of "medicine" to survive or like a vehicle needs to be topped off every three hundred miles. How effective can we really be when we need constant doses of motivation to continue pressing forward? What happens when that motivation doesn't come? Being self-powered doesn't mean we can't benefit from motivation, but we don't require it. We are able to operate in the absence of these hard-hitting dopamine dumps and can continue working at a high capacity regardless. Being self-powered gives you control of the throttle without relying on external conditions. Once you harness that superpower, nothing is out of reach.

The Unlock

The beginning of an ultramarathon sometimes feels like a bunch of friends going on an excursion or adventure like a camping trip, but it quickly evolves into an opportunity to learn a lot about yourself and your strengths and weaknesses. That's one of the reasons I encourage people to sign up for running events like Last Man Standing, an ultra, or a marathon distance race. Doing hard things on a regular basis will change your life. It doesn't have to be running related, but like Steve Magness describes in his book *Do Hard Things*, "Running is a sport where you are alone in your head navigating immense levels of discomfort. Running and similar tests of endurance provide the perfect backdrop for studying toughness."

As my crew and I waited for the noon race start time, something I had never experienced before, it was nice to set up our base camp with everything we needed. Normally, these races begin before the sun rises. The weather was ideal, and we had good access to the start and finish lines. Since BPN announced that we were going to be a sponsor for Last Man Standing, there were people from the community who signed up for this race. BPN was well-represented; all around me were "Go One More" and "Prove Yourself Right" slogans on apparel and signage. We set up our two tents and were fully prepared with all the food, extra crew members, and staff we needed.

As we were setting up, I noticed a runner and his wife at a nearby campsite. I knew the man since we followed each other online. Everybody was assigned a site, and ours looked as if we were ready to stay there for months, but this couple didn't even have a tent. All they brought was a blanket and some food. I typically take the over-prepared approach because I believe in the saying "If you fail to plan, you plan to

fail." When I first noticed them, I could tell they were arguing about something. With the sun beating down on us and
the temperature rising, we decided to walk over to them and
ask if they wanted to join us.

"Come over and use our tent and food—whatever you
need," we offered. They were reluctant but decided to come
over to our site.

I was sitting there with everybody else, joking around
and having fun because you have to keep it light for ultras.
It's not sustainable to be a hard-ass for twenty-four hours.
But when I looked over to see the runner we had invited over
with this wife, you could tell they were both in a bad mood.
In fact, I noticed a coldness that drifted in with them as soon
as they came to our tent. They weren't warm and friendly at
all. The wife looked frustrated the entire time. I could tell by
the look on her face that she didn't want to be there. And to
be honest, I didn't blame her. When I saw this guy, her husband, I knew he was overtrained, and he was already beat
down before the race had even started.

All I heard him say was a series of complaints: "My legs
hurt . . . I can't keep any food down . . . this sucks . . . I feel
sick . . . I just want to be done." It was ridiculous, and they
were bringing our energy down. I've found that, in life, there
are people who fill your cup and those who empty it. You get
to choose who is allowed to have access to your cup.

Why are you even here? I thought. *Your wife traveled out
of state to come support you, and all you're doing is being a
cancer to everybody around you.* One of the best things I've
ever heard is that "raw enthusiasm is contagious," but it also
works in the opposite direction.

It was at this moment when something clicked. It felt like a scene in a movie. I had been following this guy on social media forever, watching him prep for all of his events, competitions, and races, but when I listened to him complain like that, I suddenly had a series of questions racing through my mind.

Is this what Go One More looks like?

Is this the sort of person who has taken my message to heart?

Is this really what people think I'm telling them to do?

I knew that if that was the case, then I was doing a disservice to all the people who followed me. With all those thoughts and questions in my mind, I needed to continue running. I knew I would find clarity in the miles. I always do.

By nightfall, when I was racing in the dark, I felt right at home. Most of the runs I do are done in the dark. Every morning, I wake up between 4 and 5 AM and complete my run in time to be back home to give our daughter breakfast. I love running in the dark. It's quiet and provides me with so much solitude. I feel myself waking up with the city around me. I'm able to be incredibly focused, and this focus allows me to find clarity and reflect on my thoughts, my actions, my intentions, and everything I'm doing. My running coach, Jeff Cunningham, said it best: "People don't run to clear their heads. They run to gain clarity, which allows them to organize the thoughts, ideas, and perspectives of their mind."

That's why I sign up for things like Last Man Standing: to find clarity and organize my thoughts. Near the end of my race, I could feel it coming. For the last year of my life, I could feel something on the tip of my tongue but had been unable to find the words to summarize this gut feeling. In the last twenty-five miles of the ultra, I finally found exactly what I had been wanting to say for the past year. Go One More had evolved into something different to me, something more powerful.

I recalled a serious conversation my wife and I had a few months earlier. We were eating dinner when she opened up to me in an honest and heartfelt way.

"You know, Nick, all these things you talk about: 'Go One More' and 'Prove Yourself Right.' You apply all these things to your training and your business and your personal goals. But by the time you have exhausted all of your energy on those things, there is none left for our family."

She called me out on my crap, and just like that, my mind was blown and my heart was crushed. "You're absolutely right."

I realized I wasn't Going One More in all aspects of my life. I've always been a person who has said that family and faith are two important things, yet those are the two things I was always putting last on my list of things to get done. In reality, they never got done and were instead recycled from to-do list to to-do list. If I'm being honest with myself, I justified my lack of intentional time with my family by being the provider of the house. It was my responsibility to work, build, and create security, which awarded me a "free pass" from being the father and husband I actually wanted and needed to be.

As I ran that loop in the dark at the Last Man Standing ultramarathon, I thought back to the runner I had seen looking miserable and arguing with his wife. That wasn't what

Go One More looked like. If people thought I was telling them to do more, to keep pushing, to forget about sleep, and neglect their families, their jobs, and every other part of their lives just to keep pushing, then I was steering everyone in the wrong direction. It is my responsibility to lead by example and continue to make the difficult but right choice instead of the easy but wrong one.

Go One More is not just an action. It's an outcome. It's about intentionality.

This was the truth I had been looking for, the lock I had been hoping to open.

Go One More is about delayed gratification. We know that consistency compounds, but the work behind the consistency has to be very intentional. It has to be thought through. Just doing more of something doesn't equate to meaningful progress or growth. This sort of self-sabotage where you do more work for the sake of staying busy can lead to self-destruction. I've been there, I've seen it, and it exists all around us. Doing challenging things just to say you've done them isn't the intent. The intent is to use these challenges to unlock perspectives that help you grow into the person you are meant to be. It's about maximizing your potential.

Go One More isn't burning the candle at both ends. It's not about neglecting all your responsibilities and obligations. It's actually about honoring them. That's where the true power of Go One More exists.

I thought about that conversation with my wife, then asked myself a series of questions.

What does a life of Go One More look like?

Where is my focus? What are my priorities? My responsibilities?

Am I focused on those things?

What are my true intentions?

When I'm on my death bed, will I care about the things I accomplished?

What actually matters in life and the short amount of time we have left?

Am I fulfilling my mission?

It's easy to become consumed by things that might not move the needle in your life. To lose the clarity and vision you need. To overlook the outcome because you're so focused on the action. You can do something as hard as you can and as frequently as possible, but without intentionality, it is usually meaningless. We have to ask ourselves every day: What am I working on and why? What is the intention behind it? What is the opportunity cost associated with prioritizing those things? What am I going to unlock by focusing my time and attention on these things?

When I was in the military, each operation, no matter the mission, had a desired end state, an outcome. That outcome had a set of required conditions that achieve the strategic objective of the operation. The end state is the North Star that guides us to achievement. Without it, we are operating carelessly.

My epiphany in Last Man Standing came from a simple but profound truth about Go One More: I wasn't the last man in the race, so technically I didn't even finish it (my first DNF). But I had accomplished what I hoped to by competing in it; I unlocked a part of my mind and discovered a new truth.

Intentionality

I'll never forget the day I first read one of my favorite quotes. Jordan Utter, my creative director, is much younger than me, but he's wise beyond his years. He always has a sticky note on his desk with a different quote from something he's studying. One day while I was reviewing a video he had produced, I noticed a sticky note on the bottom of the monitor that said, "Lack of intentionality leads to a repetition of what is easiest."

Wow, I thought. *That's powerful.*

Jordan used this quote as a reminder to make the difficult, right decision instead of the easy, wrong one. Usually, the easy option lacks discipline and intention. In other words, it's easy to be lazy. We naturally want to take the path of least resistance, the path that lacks originality, innovation, discomfort, and newness. We like the predicable path that leads to safety.

If we don't lead a life with intentionality or pursue intentionality, we will just do what is easiest. Take growth, for example. Growth is challenging, but you must choose it. It doesn't just occur by chance. If you don't make the choice to grow, you will simply maintain the status quo. You will just go through the motions. Every easy path you choose to follow adds an incremental degree of separation between where you're heading and your full potential. The longer you are off course, the greater that separation becomes.

When I was in the military, we were frequently tested on our land navigation skills. We were given a compass, map, and protractor with points to locate based on an eight-digit grid coordinate. In order to successfully find your points, you needed to use terrain association, as well as a precise compass reading. If your compass reading was off by even a few degrees, it could be challenging to locate your points. And the further you walked with an inaccurate reading, the greater the degree of separation. Eventually, you would reach a point where you had been traversing so far off course that it would be nearly impossible to recover. The degree of separation between where you end up and where you intended to be is unmeasurable. Taking the easy path is a lot like following an inaccurate compass reading. If you keep taking that path, you'll be so far from achieving your goal that you'll never be able to find your way again.

Want to know what's really hard? Pausing, evaluating, taking one step back, slowing down, and leaning in with a new strategy. An intentional plan. Doing this feels like you're digressing, but you're actually preparing to make massive progress. I know this is hard because I've been in this situation many times before, and I observe people, almost daily, putting the quantity of work they do on a pedestal and ignoring the quality of their work. James Clear once said, "You're more likely to unlock a big leap in performance by trying differently than by trying harder. You might be able to work 10 percent harder, but a different approach might work 10x better. Remain focused on the core problem, but explore a new line of attack. Persistence is not just about effort, but also strategy. Don't merely try harder, try differently."

This intentionality is the starting point, the foundation

of Go One More. It's not only about the work, but more importantly the type of work and the intention behind its outcome. Just as James Clear explained, you might not need to do more and try harder, but rather take a different route to get to where you want to be.

Another way to think about this difference is by focusing on strategy instead of tactics. Strategy is the action plan that you establish to get to where you want to be. The tactics are the small action items completed within a shorter time frame that move you toward the strategic objective. If your strategy isn't working, then continuing to execute on the tactics created to support that strategy isn't going to work, either. You can keep hammering down on the tactics, but without a new strategy, you won't make any progress.

Intentional choices and decisions plant your feet on the ground and move you forward. Those forward steps are progress. I'm a visual learner, and you may be, too, so I'm going to try and paint you a picture to describe what this looks like for me. Think about an individual who keeps working on something that produces little to zero results. Imagine that they are driving a car and keep hitting the gas. They work harder and spin the wheels even faster with no incremental progress. Why? They aren't even on the ground. They are suspended in the air, and no matter how hard and fast they spin the wheels, it's impossible to move forward. The idea of this movement, however, creates an unrealistic sense of accomplishment. Their foot is pressing the pedal to the floor, but no matter how hard they press, the car doesn't budge. As soon as that same individual slows down and implements a new and intentional strategy, the car lowers to the ground.

Now, there is traction between the ground and the wheels. This new plan may require them to move slower and work less, but each step they take moves them one step closer to the result that they imagined.

Over the years, as I've interviewed many successful and talented individuals, I've learned that there is a common denominator that contributes to their success: a relentless pursuit to achieve greatness. I'm sure this is no surprise, but hard work only works when it is intentional. It works when the strategy behind the work is effective. The most successful people don't always spend the most time at work, but I can guarantee you they are hyper-focused on the right things when they are working. And once you have tasted the success that results from hard, intentional work, you'll realize it's an equation that is replicable. Unfortunately, some of these high-achieving people who make a lot of money and build businesses often neglect other parts of their lives. It's the battle between ambition and contentment, a war I have personally fought. I'm sure you have, too. This is one reason I'm writing this book—I believe we can show up for our work and fight for everything we want to achieve without sacrificing our other responsibilities and obligations in the process.

Years ago, I was listening to a podcast interview with a man who had just sold his business for $100 million.

"You spent the last two decades building this business and have sold it for $100 million," the interviewer said to the businessman. "What's the first thing you did afterward?"

"Well, after I got the money, I went to my family—my kids and my wife—and I said, 'All right, guys. Work's done. $100 million in the bank. We're going to travel the world.'"

The businessman was stunned to hear his children's reply.

"Dad . . . We don't want to travel the world with you. We haven't even *seen* you for the last two decades. You're not a part of our life. You're not the dad that we needed or wanted."

So, after years of working and toiling and grinding, the man was alone. As I listened to that, I had a haunting thought: *Is this the trajectory I'm on? Am I willing to sacrifice everything through the journey for the prize awarded at the final destination?*

Sometimes, you can be so focused on the wrong things in life, or on just *one* thing in your life, that you end up neglecting everything and everyone else. It's lost perspective. The people and things that need to be the focus of your life suddenly become only part of your life.

This book is a set of lessons I've learned—that I'm still learning—as I've explored and lived out Go One More. But here's the thing: I've learned very little through success. I've learned much more through failure. If there's a common denominator in my life, it's that I have arguably failed much more than I've succeeded. People see my successes and they attribute my entire life to them; however, I've consistently failed and refined my work through these failures (more on this in chapter 2).

Be a Key Collector

I believe we all want to discover breakthroughs. We long to find keys that unlock the mysteries in our life. But I don't think there is one key that unlocks everything. In fact, I don't think there is even a set of keys. The number of keys you can accumulate is endless if you keep placing yourself in positions to grow, experience, learn, fail, and adapt. Each opportunity you embrace creates an opportunity to achieve a key that unlocks a new perspective or idea. These keys result in confidence, maturity, and clarity.

For me, the Last Man Standing race rewarded me with a key that unlocked an entire new perspective on Go One More. I feel like I'm holding this key in my hand, and I can't wait to share it with you.

As we start this journey, ask yourself the same questions I had to answer after that conversation with my wife, Stef.

- What are your priorities and responsibilities in life?
- Do they align with the vision and mission you have for yourself and your family?
- Are you intentionally taking action that allows you to show up for these things every single day?

Let me repeat that beautiful quote I first read on Jordan's desk: "Lack of intentionality leads to the repetition of what is easiest." Here's another way to think of it: the lack of intentionality can lead you to repeatedly be overworked but underachieving. Taking action to work toward greatness is honorable, but when you don't have an intention behind it, the greatness will never be achieved.

As they say, comparison is the thief of joy. It's really easy these days, especially with social media, to observe the people in your social ecosystem who are constantly doing something and feel bad because they're always on the move, staying up late and waking up early. But just because they're doing all these things does not mean they're progressing in life. As I said, spinning your wheels doesn't mean you're making forward progress.

I don't want to be the guy dragging his miserable wife to another race she doesn't want to be involved with. And I definitely don't want to be the man who builds his business and brand only to then realize years later that he's neglected all the other aspects of his life in order to get there.

In my pursuit of greatness, I don't want to be the last man standing.

Chapter Two

BE CONSISTENTLY GOOD INSTEAD OF OCCASIONALLY GREAT

"Making a choice that is 1 percent better or 1 percent worse seems insignificant in the moment, but over the span of moments that make up a lifetime, these choices determine the difference between who you are and who you could be."

—James Clear, *Atomic Habits*

n 2014, I sat in my apartment in Belton, Texas, knowing something had to change. At that point in my life, I only had $500 to my name. All the money I was making in the Army was getting reinvested back into the company I had started two years earlier, just to keep it alive. Everyone around me who noticed my business's failure justified my lack of growth by telling me it took three years for a business to take off. At first, I bought into this explanation, but eventually, I saw it for what it was: an excuse. I couldn't afford employees, outsourced marketing, or digital advertising agencies. There was no option other than to be a one-man show. I knew what I had to do, but I was afraid to do it. I needed to get on YouTube and start making videos to promote the brand. I had to put the responsibility on myself and take ownership of the business's success or failure. YouTube was the perfect platform to share my story, document the process, and build a community through shared beliefs and values.

The problem was I had already done that. Twice.

My first video was just me talking into the camera about myself and Bare Performance Nutrition. And it received a lot of criticism.

"You're doing it wrong," someone wrote.

"SO AWKWARD," another comment said.

"Just another fitness channel . . ."

I quickly deleted the YouTube channel. A few months later, I did the same thing. I filmed a video, uploaded it, got hate, and then deleted the channel.

Now it was 2014, and I had no other option. There was nothing else to lose. I started the company by taking out a $20,000 loan with the military-associated bank USAA. It was a great deal for newly commissioned Army officers. There were no payments for the first eighteen months and a low interest rate, but I only had $500 left. The entirety of the loan went to buying inventory for the company's first production order.

I had to make this work. In the famous words of Julius Caesar, "If you want to take the island, burn the boats." So I went out and spent the rest of my money on a real camera to document my experience in the military, fitness training, and building BPN.

Burn the Boats

This was a pivotal moment in my life where I learned the tremendous value of going all in. Fitness YouTube channels were newer to the scene in 2014 with tons of opportunity. As I sat in my apartment with my first camera about to film my first real video, I was scared. I didn't want to be on camera. I didn't know what I was doing. But I knew I had to do it because I couldn't afford to pay anyone else to do it for me. So I started. If not me, then who?

If you're going to be consistent about something, then you're going to have to be brave enough to start. That's the difference between having confidence and having courage. Confidence is the belief in one's self. Many people have the confidence that one day they may build the life they want and accomplish the goals they dream of, but without action, those dreams remain dreams. Courage is the action. It's the first step. Without courage, you will only be a dreamer living in the clouds, thinking about what could be.

After posting the video, I got hate just like before, even with my fancy new camera. But this time, I weathered the storm and got through it. This time, I said, "Screw it," and left the video up. I've been making YouTube videos consistently since that fateful day in 2014. To date, I have uploaded 943 videos with 164 million views, and nine years after having the courage to take the first step, that channel has surpassed one million subscribers.

I've had seasons of fast growth and seasons of slow growth. There have been times when I've been creatively inspired and other times when I didn't have any desire to pick up a camera. I've experienced tremendous feedback from viewers and soul-crushing criticism. Through the highs and lows of documenting my life, building a business, and leading a team—all while starting a family and serving in the military—I never allowed myself to take my foot off the gas. At certain times, I've accelerated faster than others, but I kept the momentum moving forward. The consistency of those daily choices over a decade has changed my life. By focusing on being consistently good, you can achieve greatness. The goal isn't to maintain one-hundred miles per hour for your entire lifetime. That's impossible. Instead, the goal is to never let off the gas, even if you can only maintain five miles per hour for certain segments. No matter what, keep moving forward.

Sometimes at night, when I'm lying in bed, I scroll through the hundreds of videos I have filmed, edited, and uploaded to my channel over the years. I cringe watching some of the oldest ones. I was so naïve and ignorant about how challenging the journey would be, but that was the best part. I didn't know what I was getting myself into. There was an unknown to the path I was walking (to be honest, it felt like I was sprinting), and I was all in. I've made countless mistakes along the way, gotten close to running out of money more times than I'd like to admit, and ran myself into the ground, both physically and mentally, but I never quit. That's what I'm most proud of.

You don't need my permission, or anyone else's for that matter, but I urge you to give yourself some grace. I wish I would've done that for myself earlier on, because aiming for perfection held me back and slowed me down. For the last couple years, I have been resurfacing some of my early YouTube videos and sharing them with our team and audience. The video footage is painful to watch as I trip over my words, stutter through sentences, and try to find the balance of proper camera eye contact throughout the video. What did I learn through that journey? We all start somewhere, and that somewhere is zero. You can't expect to have all the answers or be at your best when you're first getting started, but you can improve. You should improve. You have to improve.

Consistency Beats Talent

Here's the thing about consistency: you don't have to be born with it. We all know what it's like to see someone with a natural talent for something. I've always been the poster child for average. Of course, my mom will argue with that, but

I will fight it all day. Pure talent is not what brought me to this point in my life. It was the compounding effect of being consistently good over the course of a decade. There is a very powerful potential you can leverage when you show up and put in the work day after day, year after year.

When I was young, I dreamed of becoming a professional baseball player. If not the pros, then at least play competitively at a Division I school. Neither happened. I grew up playing sports with guys who were God-gifted athletes. From the moment they touched the ball, they were throwing ninety-mile-per-hour heaters and catching game-winning touchdowns. I was athletic, played on varsity teams, and could keep up, but engaging in sports after high school was not in my cards. Why? I didn't apply the sustained effort to experience the success I wanted. That's the honest truth. Did I have the raw talent to get there? Maybe, maybe not, but I didn't want it bad enough, so I didn't try hard enough. I liked the idea of playing sports in college or professionally, but I wasn't willing to accept what I needed to do to get there. Talent will get you started, but it can only take you so far. There is a point on an XY axis of a graph where the consistent, hard-working individual surpasses the one who relies solely on talent. You are either born with natural talent or you're not. Consistency, however, is a choice. It's that one thing that you are in direct control over.

I didn't realize that consistency was my superpower until a couple of years ago when one of my friends turned to me and said, "Nick, you're one of the most consistent people I've ever met." It made me think. *Yeah, I guess I am pretty consistent.* But there wasn't a day I could remember when

I consciously stopped and thought, *From this day forward, thou shall be more consistent* (in my most stoic and powerful voice). I wish more of life's revelations unfolded that way. This was an adaptation, natural selection at its finest.

What has separated me from others and allowed me to reach the success levels I have is that I've chosen to be consistent. Consistency is the foundation of everything I do. This hasn't necessarily always been the case, but once I realized the power of consistency, I turned it into my competitive advantage.

During some of the toughest years of building my business, I realized the power of consistency. There wasn't one event that changed the trajectory of the company. Change and success were made slowly. I showed up every day to solve problems, identify opportunities, and be a student in the school of hard knocks. This is what I truly excel in. This mentality is why tomorrow morning, my alarm will go off at 4:20 AM, and even though staying in my warm bed next to my wife and snoozing for two more hours before our kids wake up sounds much better, I'll still put my shoes on and go run. I'll run because consistency is a decision I can control. I don't need talent to be able to do it. And it's something *everyone* can apply to their life and build upon. I've built my brand, business, and body through consistency. Trust me, it works.

Progressive Overload

You don't have to have talent to be consistent, but you do have to be consistent in order to succeed at anything in life.

Now, I would be doing you a disservice by failing to mention the second layer of consistency: progressive overload. Being consistent has the power to transform your life, but if life were a lemon, my goal would be to squeeze every ounce of juice from it. (That's turning lemons into lemonade.) You may have heard about progressive overload when it comes to increasing your fitness. To keep progressing toward your fitness goals, your training must be modified to increasingly overload the muscular, cardiovascular, and central nervous systems. If you want to get stronger, you can't expect strength to develop by performing the same movement with the same weight for the same number of reps and sets over the course of years and years and years. You will plateau. Growth will cease. Just as much as you are in control of choosing to be consistent, you must also choose to apply greater stress on your mind and body over time. Stress stimulates adaptation, and adaptation facilitates growth.

You know that guy in the gym who does the same workout every other day with the same exercises and methods of execution? Don't get me wrong—he may be the most consistent person in the gym, but I can guarantee that he won't get any stronger unless he makes changes to his training routine. Consistency is the foundation of success. You can't negotiate with consistency, but in order to keep growing and improving, you must apply progressive overload.

This technique does not only apply to fitness, but every other aspect of our lives. The gains we experience from strength training and cardiovascular conditioning happen from our bodies' response to stress. While you may think of stress on the body as a bad thing, it's actually essential to stimulate growth. Our body responds to stressors and creates adaptations so it is prepared to respond more efficiently the next time it happens.

As we pursue greater challenges in life, we are guaranteed to experience resistance, obstacles, hardship, and stress. It is inevitable. Instead of viewing these situations as negatives, a shift in perspective can shine some light on their positives. I've witnessed people turn down life-changing opportunities because the fear of failure was too great, but that failure could have actually been the overload that pushed them forward. Sometimes progressive overload isn't an obvious and intentional choice; rather, it is an event or experience that happens to us. How we respond in these scenarios can determine the strength of the resulting adaptation.

This is one of the reasons we should continue setting goals that are just beyond our realistically achievable grasp. Those goals may feel impossible in the moment, but everything is impossible if we don't ever try. The theory and practice of progressive overload trains our minds and bodies to adapt and improve. Each incremental exposure has the ability to make us a little bit stronger.

In 2016, we signed our first warehouse lease to continue building BPN. Before this, my brother and I were operating the entire business out of my 1,300-square-foot house. That first warehouse was six thousand square feet and felt massive to us at the time. Three years later, the business had grown about 230 percent, but we were still comfortable in our current warehouse space. Comfortable is what scared me. I didn't want to be comfortable. Comfortability kills momentum. I wanted to be just the right amount of uncomfortable because I knew that is what stimulates growth. I needed a stressor to push me.

Despite the advice from many trusted friends, advisors, and family members, I signed a lease for a new warehouse that was about ten thousand square feet. I knew we didn't need that much space at the time, but I also knew it would force me to make decisions that would scale the business. That additional space and rent was a healthy stressor that pushed me to do more, be better, and continue pursuing growth. That choice was one form of progressive overload, and we ended up growing an additional 400 percent just twelve months after moving into the new space.

Now, anyone can make irresponsible decisions that put them at risk of losing everything. Anyone can bury themselves in a workout, pull an all-nighter, or run themselves to the edge of burnout. That's not the purpose, goal, or intent of progressive overload. The goal is to strategically make decisions that facilitate consistent growth. Set that goal or milestone just a little bit further. Raise the standard and stakes a little bit higher than what feels comfortable, and then work to achieve it. This should stretch your capacity, but it shouldn't break you.

Controlled Discomfort

My running coach, Jeff Cunningham, understands talent because he has it and has seen it. He was an all-state distance runner in high school who earned a scholarship to Baylor University. During college, he was a member of the 1994

Southwest Conference championship team and earned conference honors in cross country and track as well as NCAA Academic All-America honors. His coaching career began in the high school ranks, coaching multiple state champions, national qualifiers, and NCAA scholarship athletes. Now, he coaches all distances from the mile to the marathon, including countless Boston Marathon qualifiers and multiple US Olympic Trials Marathon qualifiers. After working with Jeff for the last three years, he has helped me shave ninety-six minutes off my marathon time.

When Jeff and I talk about running, it is rarely entertained by the notion of talent. It is almost always focused on the theme of hard work and consistency.

"I always tell people that you don't have to be rolling around on the ground like a scalded earthworm to be able to say that you had a great workout," Jeff said. "In fact, I would posit that's probably not the best way to do it because then you're going to spend so much time recovering, you're going to feel like hammered crap the next day."

When you overdo a workout or overrun on a given day, you might feel so horrible that you're unable to work out or run the following day. You want controlled discomfort, Jeff said; you don't want to be completely wasted. How many times have we seen someone go out to the gym or on a run and destroy themselves, only to say, "Man, I crushed that workout!" But then they're lying on the ground for an hour after they're done, and they can't walk right for two days afterward. There is a time, place, and purpose for emptying the tank, but I promise you it's not daily or even frequently.

Jeff pointed out, "If we get mildly uncomfortable

repeatedly in a controlled manner, week after week, month after month, it builds this massive aerobic system. It's like doubling the number of streets and highways in your city and creates the ability to deliver so much more to its intended destination. And that's what we're doing physiologically.

"Let's just be consistently good. Let's show up. Let's understand the parameters of the workout. Let's be passionate about investment in the process and sticking to the plan, and be passionate about watching the fitness creep in almost insidiously. It's like plate tectonics; it just slowly creeps in. And then suddenly, you wake up on race day and it's like, *Wow, I put in some amazing training! I'm ready.* That's the key."

Even though Jeff was talking about the idea of being consistently good instead of occasionally great through the lens of distance running, it can be applied to other aspects of life as well. Instead of showing up and performing at an exceptional level on rare occasions, you will go much further by showing up and performing to standard on a regular and consistent basis. There will be some instances where it's better to hold back a little bit and leave some in the reserve tank so you can show up the next day with the same level of intensity. While those days won't seem to move the needle in the success of your life, over the course of years, the effect of compounding consistency will result in transformational progress.

Being consistently good instead of aiming toward the occasionally great requires intentionality and discipline. It feels good to hit the home run, catch the game-winning pass, score the big business deal, or stand on a stage to receive a career-defining award, but that's not the everyday. The everyday isn't glamorous or driven by these occasionally great, significant life events. The reality is the everyday moves us toward these celebrations. Being occasionally great is the result of the non-glamorous work that we hammer on a consistent basis.

Sharpen Your Axe

I was listening to a sermon by Pastor Erwin McManus in which he described his experience as a lumberjack when he was younger. Erwin was paid by weight for the number of trees he cut down, so there was an incentive to work hard and fast. There were a few younger lumberjacks like him, but they were mostly surrounded by older, less athletic, and less jacked gentlemen, as he described. While sizing up the younger, stronger guys against the elders, it seemed pretty obvious who would be making more money at the end of the day, but he was proven wrong.

The older guys chopped down more trees at the end of each workday, took more breaks, and made more money. How? They had their axes sharpened daily and rested during this time. "If the axe is dull and its edge unsharpened, more strength is needed," Erwin said. In order to keep your edge, you must continue to sharpen your axe because you cannot continue to improve as long as it's dull. The key is to show up with sharpened tools and resources, but in order to do that, you must be consistent with the intentional decisions you make. Each choice we choose to pursue or decline leads us in a different direction. Be sharp. Stay sharp.

I've always been turned off by the "grind" mentality. It never resonated with me. To "grind" means to put hard work on a pedestal. The "grind" is unsustainable, it's dull, and it's inconsistent. The hardest workers I know aren't out there "grinding." The level of work they consistently perform is sharp, intentional, and held at an extremely high standard. It's not an exception. I respect and value hard work more than many things in life, but it's not meant to be glorified as if it's a noun attached to your identity. It's a verb. Tim Grover describes this beautifully in his book *Winning:* "Everyone talks about 'the grind.' Well, you can grind and grind and grind, and what's left at the end? Dust. Grinding deforms, it obliterates. Excellence is about sculpting. When you sculpt, you strategically remove parts you don't need, the elements that get in the way. It's the equivalent of not just working hard but working smart."

I share these stories with you because I used to aim for occasional greatness and fail to be consistently good. I've experienced declines in my athletic performance, business dealings, relationships, and personal happiness because my axe was dull. I thought applying more force or "grinding" would overcome the dullness, but it never did. Being consistently good allows you to show up with a clear head and sharp mind. I didn't pass the US Army Ranger School with one good leadership evaluation. I didn't run a two-hour-and-thirty-nine-minute marathon from one good workout. I didn't build an eight-figure business overnight with one effective marketing strategy. All of my accomplishments are the result of consistent hard work over long periods of time with an inability to accept defeat. That's what happens when you keep showing up and chipping away at something.

You can't change your life overnight. All of the things you have to do in between where you are right now and where you want to be probably feels overwhelming. I get it. But it starts with the courage to take the first step. You build the life you want, brick by brick. If you apply consistency to that action, then you will be in a better place in five or ten years. But you have to be consistent and disciplined. Sounds simple, right? Of course. But here's the thing: it's not easy.

Simple Versus Easy

If we want to be successful at anything we set out to achieve, the first trait we need to build upon is consistency. It's the foundation to achieving greatness, accomplishing our goals, and building the life we hope to create. The more responsibilities, tasks, and processes we add to our lives, the harder it is to maintain consistency with any of them, so it's important that we simplify many parts of our lives so we can accomplish our goals.

Being consistent is simple, but it's not easy. Simple and easy aren't synonyms. Like a lot of people, I used to use those two words interchangeably, but I've discovered that they are very different. Simple is focused. It is often reducing the amount of things we are working on. It's turning down a hundred good ideas so we can say yes to the one great one. That process and those decisions can be some of the hardest, but also the most transformational. We shouldn't be afraid of simple. But we should be afraid of easy.

During a conversation for my podcast with Bedros Keuilian, we discussed the number one thing that holds most people back from reaching their full potential: the story we tell ourselves, one that is partly true. For some people, this stems from our childhood experiences, the environment in which we were raised, and the failures and lies we believe about who we are. This lack of confidence has the ability to destroy who we could be—it's self-sabotage.

"What I found through my life experience is that you wind up looking for evidence to reinforce that story throughout the rest of your life," Bedros said. "Why you're not lovable, why you're not smart, why you can't lose weight, why you should be broken your whole life. And so the moment you can realize that 'I can take back the pen that I've empowered others with who have been writing in my book of life. And I can start rewriting my story from this day forward,' then you start looking for evidence for your new story. I *can* be lean. I *can* create financial freedom. I *can* be loved. I'm not just to be thrown away. I don't have to be in an abusive relationship. But it's about self-empowerment. It's really about taking that pen back and rewriting your story because I think, we could all agree, until you die, you certainly have thousands of pages of blank pages left in your book of life. It's time to start writing your current story and not so much living out the past story that you had."

I asked Bedros if he thought it was easy to go from

telling yourself one story one day to changing the narrative the next day.

"So it's simple, not easy," Bedros said. That's because it's a simple concept to understand, but it's difficult to act on "because our brains are so good at creating neural pathways to reinforce things. So for years, if you keep going and finding abusive relationships to then justify why you should be abused, because your subconscious mind still believes that you're not worthy of love and respect, then you have to create new patterns of life. You have to create a new neural pathway. This is why we talk about habits, right? This is why we talk about how small micro habits become lifelong habits that are hardened and create a pattern of life. Is it easy? No, it is simple, but it does take a good amount of time, maybe working with a therapist, maybe doing the deep work, journaling your thoughts, feelings, and emotions. Why do I feel this way? Where is it coming from? But oftentimes people are too busy distracting themselves, escaping from the reality either through social media or binge-watching television or vices like alcohol or pornography or weed or gambling, whatever the thing might be. And so they never take time to just sit with themselves and go, *What is going on with me, and how can I actually rewrite my story?* And then doing the work to do that. Like anything else, it takes time and effort, but the outcome that it produces can shape a brand-new life."

Simple, not easy.

Sometimes it's easy to try to change others, yet it's difficult to try to change ourselves. Habits are hard to break, especially when we are having to literally rewrite our story. Yes, the world is simple. A lot of the things that we experience, do, or want to do are simple. But just because they might be simple doesn't mean they are easy.

Simple used to scare me. I once thought that making things simple would make me look uneducated. It would make me appear like I was taking the path of least resistance, and we know that the stimulants of resistance build strength through adaptation. So, to compensate, I would overcomplicate everything and anything. I did this to make myself feel smarter and look smarter to people around me. It took many years to realize that by avoiding simple (not easy), I was making things harder for myself and others. Not only was I an ineffective communicator, but I was also an ineffective leader.

Making things simpler does not mean you're making them easier. Embracing simplicity helps you become more effective at everything you do for yourself, your family, and the people you lead. Simplifying allows you to be more focused, with greater clarity on what matters and how it's achieved. Simplifying allows you to be more consistent. I have had the opportunity to work under and alongside some amazing leaders, and I've learned from their successes, failures, confidence, and insecurities. Oftentimes, some of the most incompetent "leaders" will overcomplicate the work to manipulate you into thinking you aren't on their level yet or you aren't smart enough to understand their reasoning. It took me many years to realize this foolish tactic because the greatest, most competent, and most effective leaders will simplify their work. They don't take the easy path, but they choose the simplest route for the team's ability to execute flawlessly.

Let me share a very personal and very real example with you about the concept of simple not easy. When I was fourteen years old, I had a severe eating disorder where I was starving myself. Now, I would consider myself a "bigger-boned" teenage boy, but not overweight, unhealthy, or someone you would think needed to lose a few pounds. To this day, I can't explain to you why I became obsessed with becoming thinner, but it was truly an obsession. My entire day revolved around eating less and working out more. The only thing I can really pinpoint it down to is that I wanted to have some sort of level of control in my life, so losing weight was one part of my life that I could control and manipulate. My parents didn't obsess over our food choices, but we were raised on a well-balanced diet. We ate fresh, local food, but also enjoyed going out for dinner, hosting BBQs, and grabbing a pizza after sports practice. Nothing in my early childhood led to an obvious explanation of developing an eating disorder, but it happened.

My obsession with food and losing weight started with eliminating certain "bad foods," like cookies, soda, and sweet treats. Over a few quick months, it gradually turned into a full-blown problem. At the time, my school lunch consisted of a turkey and cheese sandwich, a bag of chips, an orange, and a bottle of water. First, I got rid of the bag of chips, then a few weeks later, I got rid of the orange. A few weeks later, I cut off the edges of the bread. Then I got rid of the bread altogether. I eventually got to a point where I was just drinking the bottled water and eating a slice of turkey. If

I went to my next class feeling hungry, I would think to myself, *Win!* The longer I did this, the skinnier I got. I remember touching my hip bone every day, multiple times a day during this time. After months of starving myself, I could feel my hip bone protruding through my skin—another win in my teenage head.

These eating habits coincided with excessive workouts. At night, while my parents were busy cleaning up after dinner and watching television, I would go down to the basement to jump rope while wearing sweatpants and two sweatshirts, then swing my baseball bat a million times. Just to sweat. Later on, I'd take a hot bath and then do a couple hundred sit-ups. When our family would go out to dinner, I would binge beyond control, eating everything in sight plus everyone's leftovers, and then feel sick for the next couple days. Things got to a point where I was very fatigued, and my stomach began to hurt. One Saturday morning, I was so exhausted I couldn't even get out of bed to go to my baseball game. It was a level of fatigue that was much greater than missing out on a few hours of sleep or running myself into the ground. It felt like I was dying, and I probably was.

Knowing something was wrong, my mom took me to Hershey Medical Center to figure out what was happening. They ran all sorts of tests on me. At one point, they thought I might have gotten a tapeworm from a recent vacation. Then, they thought I had celiac disease, so they put me on a gluten-free diet. Nothing seemed to be working, and everybody was puzzled. Everybody except me. I wasn't trying to waste people's time or medical resources, but I was embarrassed by my problem. I was ashamed.

For a year, the doctors and my family tried to figure out why I was losing so much weight at such a significant rate and why I was so tired all the time. I was fourteen years old, so I should have been thriving with too much energy, running up and down the streets, pumping with all the testosterone my body was producing at this age, yet instead, I was starving myself. I was essentially killing myself.

One day, when my mom picked me up at school to drive me to the Hershey Medical Center, I went in assuming we would be doing just another routine test. Maybe they'd take my blood or put a scope down my throat to check on my stomach. At this point, anything was fair game. I played along nicely. While driving in, we always turned left to go to the ER, but on this day, we turned right. As we pulled up to one building, I saw a sign that read "Eating Disorder Clinic."

Oh, crap, they know.

After walking into the building, a doctor sat down with me.

"We know what you've been doing, Nick," the doctor said. "You've been starving yourself."

My world was shattered. It felt like my brain was a collection of papers that someone just threw into the wind. So many thoughts flooded my mind so quickly that I couldn't think straight. I could no longer make up any excuses. Instead, I just broke down and began to cry. I had been caught. I was embarrassed. Everyone knew I was starving myself. For over a year, I had wasted my parents' and my doctors' time. People were so worried about me and had invested a lot of emotional energy into trying to help me, and I was doing it to myself the entire time.

The solution was actually very simple. All I had to do was eat more food.

That's all I had to do to fix my problem: consume more calories. Put more substance in my mouth, chew it, and digest it. Then I would get better. I would feel better. My energy would come back, and so would the weight. My performance would increase, and I'd be able to get out of bed easier in the morning.

Simple, right?

It was one of the hardest things I ever had to do in my life. It took years to get better and rebuild a healthy relationship with food. Even to this day, my eating disorder still gets triggered at different intersections of my life. It's something I will live with forever. It's a part of me that is dormant for long periods of time and then awakened out of nowhere, typically when I feel like I'm losing control.

The solution was so simple, but just because something is simple does not mean it is easy.

Choosing Simple Is a Sign of Intelligence

Allegedly, Albert Einstein once said, "Everything should be made as simple as possible, but not simpler." The irony is that the quote itself was simplified from the original statement he gave during a lecture in Oxford:

"It can scarcely be denied that the supreme goal of all theory is to make the irreducible basic elements as simple and as few as possible without having to surrender the adequate representation of a single datum of experience."

The former paraphrased quote is often used as an appeal to make a subject as easy as possible to understand, but not so easy that it becomes meaningless. It is an art to condense material yet not lose its substance. As the great jazz composer Charles Mingus once said, "Making the simple complicated is commonplace; making the complicated simple, awesomely simple, that's creativity."

Albert Einstein believed there were five ascending levels of intelligence: smart, intelligent, brilliant, genius, and the highest level, simple. I appreciate this mindset, and since learning about it, I have made it a goal of mine to try and simplify as much of my life as possible, especially in the way I articulate my messages. I never want to be like the guy our team at BPN talked to on the phone one day. After the call, we were all mentally and emotionally exhausted. One of my team members explained the experience perfectly: "That guy just said a thousand words without saying anything."

That really stuck with me. How many times have we tried to get a message across, and in the process, we have spoken a thousand words or taken a thousand actions or created a thousand steps without actually creating or doing or saying anything? Sharing information is important, but we don't want to overcomplicate our lives. It takes a lot of creativity to simplify the complicated. This was something I wish I understood before my first speaking event.

Right after I got out of the Army, I was asked to speak at an event in Dallas, Texas, for people transitioning out of the military into civilian life. I was supposed to talk about this transition as well as how I built my business and what I learned. Simple! (Or so I thought.) I've been telling this story forever. But this time, I forgot that, though it may be simple, it wouldn't be easy. Most of the time, I do a lot of prep, but in this case, I really didn't even think about it. I didn't take the time to consider who I was talking to or the intent of my speech. I didn't have a goal for what I was going to say, nor did I have a plan for how it was going to impact the people in the audience. I didn't prepare to tell my story in the best way possible.

When I finally walked up on the stage and saw all the people in the audience, a feeling of dread fell over me. *I should have prepped.* With all their eyes on me, I really had no clue what I was going to talk about. I had planned to just tell my story, but they didn't know who I was, nor did they care about my biography. They just wanted to know how the message I was sharing was going to positively impact them. I froze for a second, then just started talking. The talking turned into spewing and rambling. I went from point A to point D to point B to point F to point C to point Z. I was all over the place and overcomplicated everything I was trying to get out. I said a thousand words without really saying anything, and after the speech was over, I walked off the stage mentally and emotionally exhausted, knowing I should have prepped and not knowing if anybody took anything from my talk.

A few weeks later, I was sent input from the audience feedback cards. One feedback card read, "Great story but not relatable to anything that I'm experiencing or going through right now." It felt like a dagger went through my chest. I needed to be a more effective leader and communicator. I needed to learn how to simplify my message. When you overcomplicate things like I did (and still do), and when you're not confident in what you're doing, you tend to start talking and moving in circles. If you're really clear and confident, and you simplify your plan and process, it's effective. Complicated is so often ineffective.

When I was in the Army, we used the acronym KISS: Keep It Simple, Stupid. It can be applied to anything—effective communication, good leadership, or a compelling message or story. Again, it's not always easy to do, but we still have to keep it simple, stupid. We all are going to end up overcomplicating something (or everything) in our lives. But our goal should be to be uncommon with creativity. You don't want an easier life; you want a simpler life. An easy life is one set on cruise control, on autopilot.

In order for us to make life simpler, we must get creative. You won't find the answers in a textbook, and the "how-to" guide doesn't exist (at least, I haven't come across it yet). It's very common to approach creativity with a "more is better" approach, but I would encourage you to do the opposite. What parts of your life can you reduce or eliminate? How can you narrow your focus and go deeper on those things? That exercise of identifying and removing is (and should be) difficult. It should be easy, but in order to show up consistently and in a meaningful way for the parts of your life that matter, you have to create the conditions for a more simple life.

The Hard Right over the Easy Wrong

For years, I have preached about choosing the "hard right over the easy wrong," meaning you make the right decision even though it's difficult instead of making the wrong choice because it's the easy one, the one of least resistance and effort. These intentional decisions result in delayed gratification. They result in a consistent positive return. They result in greatness.

It's easy to wake up early in the morning, look outside at the freezing rain, and decide to skip your workout—a commitment you made to yourself and the standard you have set. But it's much harder to see the freezing rain, get your gear on, and head out the door anyway. That's the choice we all have: the easy wrong of staying inside or the hard right of getting out there and battling the elements. The hard decision is usually the right one. It's not as sexy, doesn't get all the likes or attention you would expect, and it often takes longer to fulfill.

The hard right is morally correct, ethical, and something you will be proud of. When you choose the hard right, you can rest easy at night. The easy wrong, however, often leads you to a road of clean up, distrust, and a short-lived "riding high" moment before it all comes to a destructive halt.

There are extreme examples of choosing the easy wrong, such as lying, stealing, and cheating. Businessmen and women who have lied to their clients and forged financial documents have been sent to jail for years for the crimes they have committed, but that time spent in confinement can't measure up to the guilty conscience they have to live with for the rest of their life. At some point in their career, they decided to steer the wheel away from the hard right and ultimately paid the consequences.

These extreme cases of choosing the easy wrong over the

hard right can end up ruining lives, but there are less serious choices we experience daily. While they may not put us in jail, they do add up and create habits that spill over to other parts of our lives. Allowing dirty dishes to pile up in the sink for our spouse to clean up, leaving our grocery cart in the middle of the parking lot, and letting our dog poop in someone else's yard and pretending we didn't see it are all examples of the easy wrongs that occur every single day. Many people don't think much of them, but they instill habits and compound into something larger and more destructive. Those are the easy things we can change right now, but we also need to choose hard challenges to pursue in the process.

When discussing consistency with YouTuber Chris Williamson on my podcast, he talked about the importance of doing hard things: "One of the most common traits among the high performers that I speak to is they are electing to put themselves through hard things very frequently." It's a way to build confidence, to repeatedly tell yourself, *I can do this.*

"Consistency won't guarantee success," he said, "But not being consistent will guarantee that you won't be successful. And not electing to do hard things very regularly would probably be a close second."

The truth is hard choices are inescapable. Some challenges we choose, and others are simply factors of life. There is great value to be gained from choosing the hard right over the easy wrong. It will kick-start your personal and professional development and teach you lessons that you never would have learned otherwise. Two specific decisions to choose something hard in my life have gotten me where I am today: joining the military and starting BPN. Neither of these have been easy, but out of these hardships have come some of the greatest and most rewarding moments of my life.

Here are some truths to remember about choosing the hard right:

- **"Hard" is a relative term.** What's hard for you may not be hard for someone else, and vice versa. We should avoid comparing what is hard in our lives to what others are facing. You can choose the path of resistance and what it looks like to welcome hard things into your life. These hardships don't have to be extreme. You can embrace and adapt to challenges just beyond your current comfort zone. As you conquer challenges, what used to be hard will become manageable, what used to be manageable will become routine, and best of all, what used to be unimaginable will become achievable.

- **Choosing the hard right leads you to a better life.** Better doesn't mean easier, but taking the path of the hard right will help you create better opportunities. Hardships will ultimately expose your weaknesses, giving you a roadmap of your most important growth areas. When you choose the hard right, life offers direct insights into lessons that need to be learned and experiences you need to gain. Growth requires stress, and hard things are signs that you are moving in the right direction.

- **Make it a standard.** You have the power to decide. Will you embrace hard things in life, or will you sit back and wait for a level of growth that will never come? This is an important question to consider because growth and progression are about much more than yourself. The more you choose hard things, the greater the possibility that you will positively influence the lives of others. And it all starts with a choice.

When I talk about choice, I'm not just talking about choosing to run a marathon or not or start a business or not. I'm talking about any choice. I'll share an example of a night out when my daughter Charli was almost one year old. Before she was born, my wife Stef and I used to go out to eat and see families having dinner. Their kids would make a mess, and they would walk out of the restaurant, leaving that mess for the servers and bussers to clean up. I've always said the way you do one thing is the way you do everything, and I knew I didn't want to be someone who doesn't take responsibility for their actions, including their own mess. So I watched those families walk out and told myself that I would always clean up after myself and my family when we go to dinner.

So one particular night when Stef, Charli, and I were out to eat with my brother and his wife, Charli made a mess like she does at every dinner. As we were wrapping up dinner, I got on my hands and knees and cleaned up the mess like I always do. At the table next to us, there was a family of five with three children between the ages of four and ten. The dad watched me with astonishment as I picked up food off the floor.

"Hey, man," he said to me, "you don't do that when you go to restaurants. The reason you take your family out is so you don't have to clean up after yourself."

"No, our family doesn't do that," I said in a friendly way as I continued to clean up after myself and my daughter.

When I got back in my seat, the manager came over and gave me a free margarita because of what I did. Now, I didn't clean up after myself because I wanted a margarita, nor did I think I deserved one. I did it because it was the right thing to do, the hard right thing. The fact that he gave me a margarita showed that I was the exception because so many people choose the easy wrong.

Is choosing the hard right over the easy wrong the norm in your life? Remember that the way you do one thing is the way you do everything. Decide to consistently clean up your mess, take ownership and accountability, and be an example for your family and the people around you. *That* is choosing the hard right over the easy wrong.

Casual Sloppiness

When I first heard the term "casual sloppiness," I loved it just as much as I disliked it. I love it because it describes the way so many people approach their life and work. It's audibly interesting. I dislike it because of how accurately it describes the standard in which people do things. It's disappointing. We should all strive for excellence instead of perfection, but in all cases, we should avoid casual sloppiness. Casual sloppiness is laziness. It is careless. It lacks discipline and any type of standard set by the individual or the organization they are a part of. People who operate with casual sloppiness leave a job, task, or project unfinished so when you find it, you have to re-do it, finish it, or trash it. It creates less work for the doer and more work for everyone else. It's irresponsible and selfish.

My entire life has been focused on getting things done, not perfecting them. When we get something done, we can make different iterations of it, improving and making it better each time. The goal is to strive for consistent improvement, not perfection. However, an inability to achieve perfection does not justify the excuse to execute with casual sloppiness.

Perfection does not exist. We can strive toward it, with it set as the vision of our North Star, but pure perfection is impossible. When people realize this, many of them ask themselves, "Then what is the point?" The point is progress. It is improvement. It is getting one step better to continuously evolve, grow, and adapt. The thought of perfection can scare many away from getting started in the first place, or it can hold them back from finishing what they started. A tattoo artist, for example, could work on a piece forever until it reaches what they would consider perfection, but at some point, the work needs to be done so they can move on to the next piece and keep challenging themselves. This book is something I could keep adding to, editing, and modifying over years and years, but that wouldn't do anyone any good, including myself. When you finally accept the reality that nothing is perfect, you can't allow that to change the effort you apply to your work because doing so leads to casual sloppiness.

The person who strives for the occasionally great rather than the consistently good will go above and beyond every once in a while, and when they do, it's impressive. The results are remarkable, but everything outside of that one moment is subpar. It's sloppy. But the person who chooses to be consistently good rather than occasionally great is reliable. They execute to standard. They finish what they start and don't accept anything less than what is expected. I want the consistently good individual on my team. They may not be the one who throws the Hail Mary pass once every ten games, but they make the tackles, get first downs, and protect the quarterback with every opportunity.

In the early days of building my business, I used to reference a quote by Mark Zuckerberg: "Move fast and break things." But at some point, I stopped because I realized it was encouraging people to operate with the mindset of casual sloppiness. I interpreted that quote to mean it is important to move fast but effectively, and in the process of moving quickly, you will break things that aren't willing to move with you—systems, routines, processes, models, blueprints, etc. I didn't want people to fear breaking those things, which, in my mind, facilitated a paralysis-by-analysis problem. The reality was many people took this quote as an opportunity to be sloppy with their work and ignore the standard. It created an environment that lacked intentionality, big-picture problem solving, and due diligence. People ignored the collateral damage that their decisions created and the impact on other parts of the business. I now prefer to reference the timeless saying that I learned into during my time in the military: "Slow is smooth, and smooth is fast." This quote encourages people to slow down and be thoughtful so the decisions they make and implement can facilitate faster growth, improvement, and progress.

Don't be casually sloppy. Don't rush to failure. Set the standard, hold the standard, and work toward making progress. Your work will show for it, the results will follow, and you will become a more trusted and reliable individual. While perfection may not exist, improvement does and always will. You cannot make progress if the work you are doing is sloppy with a few occasional home runs.

Consistency Compounds

I love tying the word "endurance" to the word "consistency." You can apply this not only to running but to anything in life. In order to run faster for longer distances, you have to be prepared to run slower. Trust me, when I first started logging miles, this logic made no sense to me. Running slower should only make me slower, right? Wrong. This is about building your aerobic base and foundation. When training for a marathon, I ran a lot of slow miles below my max aerobic heart rate. These runs require discipline, consistency, and patience, but they are the most important ingredients to a successful training block. Over time, this builds your aerobic capacity and endurance. These runs are sometimes the hardest. They take longer than you want them to and you know you could run faster, but fast isn't the goal—slower is.

There's no shortcut to anything in life. This might sound like common sense to you, and I'm sure you have heard it a million times before, but we all fall for the trap every once in a while. A shortcut may have worked once before, but I promise you it's not the norm. You have to log the miles, whether it's literal miles or figurative ones. It might take weeks, months, or in some cases, years. In a digital age where more and more people are gravitating toward instant rewards, I have found appreciation for delayed gratification. It's fun to go fast. Speed releases short-term endorphins and adrenaline, but it does not always result in endurance, and endurance is where you truly create the success you desire.

As you go through life, you're going to be faced with obstacles and speed bumps. There's going to be resistance—hills and headwinds, as I like to refer to them. If you have ever gone for a run or ridden a bike, you have probably experienced this. It feels like you're either running up a hill or the wind is blowing into your body, no matter what route you take or direction you head. When you hit those hills or that headwind, it's a reminder that the journey is never easy and the result is earned, never given. We have to keep pushing through those obstacles. It's not always going to be fun. In fact, it's likely going to suck. You're going to fail at times, many times. It's going to hurt. All of that is going to happen, but it's also going to build endurance. When you look back over a period of time, you will see how much progress you made because you chose to build endurance and become consistently good rather than trying to be occasionally great.

Life is a massive endurance event where if you are always aiming to be occasionally great, you're going to burn out. It's like watching inexperienced runners attempt their first marathon. They go out hard and fast at an unsustainable effort for their current conditioning. Some never make it to the finish line, and others crawl across at a pace much slower than they started. This accurately describes my first couple races.

But if you keep moving forward and remain consistently good, at a sustainable pace, you will surprise yourself by how far you can go. The key to a strong race is to consistently hit your mile splits; hold a sustainable, but hard, heart rate; consume your nutrition, hydration, and electrolytes; and lean in when it gets hard. "Consistently good" only gets better with time. It's like a fine wine or a strong investment portfolio. The growth and value compound significantly.

The best things in life are built and not bought. One of the things that makes the business I've built over the last decade of my life so unique is the community, brand loyalty, and support we receive from our committed consumers. You can't buy that. You can't spend money to acquire new customers who believe in your mission and align with your values. It takes time, trust, and value. You have to be consistent with your messaging, value proposition, and delivery.

What makes transforming your body through diet and exercise so fulfilling? It's the result of compounding consistency. Work day in and day out. You can't buy endurance or strength. You can't buy the love of your family. You can't buy the things that really matter in life. True happiness doesn't have a price tag, and anyone who tells you otherwise is lying. Focus on building the foundation of your happiness through the needs in your life, and you will experience abundant success.

I've never been the smartest, fastest, strongest, or most talented person in the room, but when I realized my ability to maintain a consistent work ethic, I knew I had found my competitive advantage. There is so much power in incremental wins. You won't see or feel them daily, but after five or ten years, you will start to realize the significant effect. For the last decade, I've been focused on stacking small incremental wins on a consistent basis.

Showing up and being consistently good creates results. Consistency compounds. Training for a marathon is hard. Building a business is hard. Being a great husband and father is hard. If you start with the expectation of succeeding right away, you are probably going to be disappointed. Consistency always wins. Show up day after day, week after week, month after month, year after year, and keep putting in that hard work because it will compound over time. That compounding consistency only gets better and better and better.

Consistency is the foundation to build everything else on.

Chapter Three

ENDURE THE PROCESS

"The journey is the reward."
— Chinese Proverb

Chadd Wright never had to run an ultramarathon to prove himself. As a kid growing up in the hills of North Georgia, Chadd dreamed of one day becoming a Navy SEAL. After failing the Physical Screening Test multiple times, he was finally able to attend boot camp, only to discover he had a pericardial cyst on his heart. He continued to pursue his goal, first by finding a surgeon who agreed to do a risky surgery on his heart, and next by building his physical fitness enough to finally join this elite team. After twelve years of serving as a team leader and master training specialist as a Navy SEAL, he retired in 2019. Since then, Chadd has become a successful business owner, entrepreneur, husband, and ultra runner. He's also become a personal friend.

Over the years, I've had some amazing conversations with Chadd—while sitting down for a podcast or going out for some runs. I've been appreciative and grateful for his mentorship and guidance. One of the things he talked about is that everything in life that facilitates growth requires a long process.

"Nobody wants to endure the process," Wright told me. "They want to settle into some mundane life. They want to settle into something that's just easy for them. That's just checking the box. They don't want to endure the process. And everything in life that forces you to grow is going to require a long and arduous process. That's in your fitness, that's in your faith, that's in your journey as a husband, as a father, as a wife, as a mother. In every aspect of your life, you've got to go through it."

Chadd came to a better understanding of what this looked like through his experience running in the Cocodona 250. He had heard about this epic ultramarathon in Arizona and was excited to participate, but deep down, it scared him. He thought about doing the race for two years before he finally registered for it. As he explained to me, one of the things that stopped him was that the race was totally outside the realm of his past experiences. But also, he couldn't bring himself to the place where he was willing to commit to the work he knew he was going to need to put in to complete the event.

"So the fact that it made me nervous, the fact that I was hesitant about it, told me something about myself," Chadd said. "Oh, man, Chadd—you're not really willing to put in the work that it's going to take to potentially finish this thing. It's telling you something about yourself. Just considering this event forced me to take this inventory of myself."

After retiring from the Navy, Chadd started the 3 of 7 Project with his brother Blake to help people become the best version of themselves. Chadd and Blake have become instrumental in training, mentoring, and inspiring others. So when it came to the Cocodona 250, Chadd realized that if he was going to continue to be an example for others, he didn't have a choice. This ultra was the perfect thing for him to lean into.

"It was making me feel the same way a lot of people that I train feel about running their first 5K. And so I had gotten to a point where I didn't feel like I could relate to many people who were just getting started anymore because I forgot what it felt like to be nervous. I forgot what it felt like to not want to put in the required amount of work to actually get it done. I forgot what it felt like to think, *Holy crap, I might not finish.*"

So the Cocodona 250 was his opportunity to do something that would bring him back to a place where he could relate to people who might just be getting started or those who weren't as far along in their journey as he was, which would enable him to be a real mentor for anyone who came out to do a rite of passage with him. It would allow him to truly help them move through it.

"One of the things I live my life by is that growth only comes through tension," Chadd said to me. "And that's in all aspects of life. Without the tension, you're actually going in reverse. So you're not even maintaining. And that is the truth. That's the God-honest truth."

That tension Chadd talked about is required maintenance. What happens to a vehicle that sits in your garage without upkeep, routine driving, and regular care? It rusts, erodes, and fails to start the longer it sits. It doesn't maintain its current condition. It breaks down without tension. We need tension in our life because without it, we erode.

Chadd knew that doing anything difficult for the first time shocks your system. The first time you run a marathon, the first time you run a hundred miler. It obliterates you. In his documentary *One Mile Out*, Chadd pushed himself and showed viewers how much he hurt both physically and mentally throughout the process. About halfway through the race, after about 120 miles, Chadd began to struggle. He had over one hundred miles left, and he couldn't wrap his mind around that fact. For the first time in a long time, he was experiencing a challenge that was breaking him down. This was a rare thing for him.

"It was such a liberating experience," Chadd told me.

Watching Chadd's Cocodona 250 documentary was inspiring on many levels, especially when he neared the end of the race. Chadd explained that when you get one mile out from the finish line, you are most likely to slip or settle for less physically and mentally. It's the last mile that counts. It's in that last mile that the greatest achievements or failures are made. And for every twenty-mile leg of the Cocodona, Chadd found the last mile to be the toughest.

"It's all just a process to get you to the last mile, and that's where you're going to experience the most growth," Chadd said. "If you keep doing the things that you know need to be done, you experience the most growth in that last mile. That's just the way you have to endure this long process."

One of the reasons I love ultramarathons is because of the distinct parallels they share with the greater experience of life. From the moment the race begins to the moment it ends, you are enduring a process. And that journey starts well before the actual race is initiated. There are hundreds of miles and countless hours you have to log in order to successfully finish the race. Of course, you can sign up for an ultra, choose not to train properly, ignore effective nutrition strategies, and just "wing it," but I think we all know how that ends. If you fail to plan, you should plan to fail. I've always said that everyone who signs up for a hundred miler dreams of crossing that finish line, but few romanticize about miles seventy, eighty or ninety. Those miles hurt. Those miles feel like they are never going to end, and each additional one feels like they are getting longer and longer. They aren't pretty, motivating, or glamorous, but they are an essential part of the process. Just like in life, there are miles we have to cover to get where we want to be. The reason crossing that finish line feels so good isn't because of the destination, but the journey—the process you endure and the growth you experience along the way.

Endurance Is the Key

In 2021, I ran the Leadville Trail 100, my first ultramarathon. It was one of the greatest experiences of my entire life. For years, I had heard of this race over and over again. The annual ultramarathon is a race over rugged trails in Leadville, Colorado, through the Rocky Mountains. In his book *Born to Run*, Christopher McDougall describes the Leadville Trail 100 as "running the Boston Marathon two times in a row with a sock stuffed in your mouth," then hiking "to the top of Pike's Peak" and doing it all over again, "this time with your eyes closed."

I had entered the lottery for the run before, but I was not selected. Fortunately, 2021 was my lucky year. The day before the race kicked off, our team was out doing a recon, scouting the course and looking at different checkpoints, when we came across an older gentleman walking past us. He might have been in his late seventies or early eighties.

"What are you guys doing up here?" he asked us. "Going to be racing tomorrow?"

"Yes, sir, I'm running," I told him.

We made small talk for a little bit before he left us with some final parting words.

"You know what the secret is to tomorrow? The secret thing that can get you across the finish line? It's this thing called . . . endurance."

He continued to explain why many of the younger, more athletic runners fail to complete the race, while the older, wiser, and potentially less fit runners succeed.

We all started laughing, thinking, *This guy's lost it!* Of course, the key was endurance. That's what an ultramarathon is all about. But as I thought about it more over time, I realized that old man was wise, that he was trying to tell us something much more than what we first took at face value.

What he was telling us was applicable to a lot more things than just a race. It wasn't just about finishing the Leadville Trail 100. Endurance is applicable to all parts of life. Your professional career. Building a family. Having kids. Marriage. Being in a relationship. Building a business. Endurance is patience. It's consistency. It's the work over a long period of time. It's wisdom.

Ultimately, he was telling us to endure the process, to embrace the journey. Yes, I was about to endure a one-hundred-mile race the next day, but running itself is a journey. Endurance isn't something you are born with; it is an ability that is built and improved through adaptation and strategic stress. If you attempt to rush the process and skip the required steps, in their required order, you can expect failure. Endurance is the key that unlocks many of the closed doors life has to offer.

I learned a lot during that one-hundred-mile race, which lasted twenty-seven hours and fifty-three minutes. To this day, I often think back to the peaks and valleys I experienced in Leadville and the lessons instilled in me during that effort. When I lined up that morning at 4 AM, I looked into the distance and the only thing I could see was mountains. It was exciting and intimidating. After the race kicked off and I was a few miles in, I couldn't help but think about what the older gentleman told me the day prior: the secret is endurance. I still didn't fully understand what he was trying to tell me, but I was about to.

The first few checkpoints felt nearly effortless, and I began to get ahead of myself a bit. I picked up my pace, passed runners as I progressed along the course, and started reminiscing about the finish line. I started visualizing the team cheering me on and imagining myself eating the sausage-and-egg breakfast burritos that were served at the coffee shop in town. My focus on the process was fading as finishing clouded my mind.

I reached mile marker thirty-eight at Twin Lakes Village in respectable time. From there, I had to climb over Hope Pass two times before returning to Twin Lakes Village to link up with my crew at mile marker sixty-two. The top of Hope Pass reached the peak elevation for the race at 12,600 feet. Coming from Texas, this was quite a shock to my system, and after returning from the brutal climbs, every inch of my body hurt. That was the moment I realized that those next thirty-eight miles to get to the finish line were going to be a fight.

My mindset and mission had to shift from thinking about celebrating after the race to each individual mile on its own. Every step, every climb, every checkpoint, and every mile had to be intentionally respected and endured. This is what the older gentleman was warning me about. Anyone can go out fast and hard, but it's the wise who endure the process and pace themselves appropriately.

I crossed the finish line of the Leadville Trail 100 with two hours and seven minutes to spare before the thirty-hour time cap. That race broke me unlike any other physical effort I had ever endured. I couldn't sleep for days afterward, I could barely walk, my body was swollen, a few toes were broken, and breathing was extremely difficult. But I learned a valuable lesson during that race. I experienced a breakthrough and unlocked a closed compartment in my mind that wouldn't have been opened otherwise. We must be willing to endure the process of life, and if we respect the process, we will be rewarded with the wisdom to achieve our greater potential.

Be Patient in Your Weakness

One of my good friends, Sally McRae, is a professional ultra runner who has won Badwater 135 and has completed the grand slam of two-hundred-mile races, which is finishing four two-hundred-plus-mile races from May to October in a given year. Those are just a few of her accomplishments. Sally is a badass athlete, entrepreneur, wife, mother, and role model.

Sally and I have had some amazing, deep conversations, and I respect her perspective on all things in life. In one of our most recent discussions for my podcast, Sally and I talked about the importance of enduring the process. She said, "You have to be patient in your weaknesses to grow." She was initially referring to a weakness in running, as she was preparing for the Western States 100, but this can be applied to every aspect of our lives.

Many of us will naturally play to our strengths, maximizing our ability and avoiding our weaknesses at all costs. Why? It's easy. Our weaknesses expose a part of us that may be an insecurity, and we want to hide that side of ourselves from others. Weaknesses also slow us down. We're forced to learn a new skill, ask for help, or search for answers, while our strengths allow us to operate with fluidity. Identifying our weaknesses also forces us to have very honest conversations with ourselves, and sometimes avoiding that internal confrontation is easier than all the work required to turn it into a strength.

Part of enduring a process is identifying our weaknesses, but the most important part is being patient with that weakness. Don't avoid it. Don't rush past it. Don't put a Band-Aid on it. Be patient and take the time to find out why it's a weakness and what is holding you back from turning it into a strength.

Building a business is a process. I have been building Bare Performance Nutrition for years. It started in my small college apartment, and now we have an eighty-thousand-square-foot central office outside of Austin, Texas. During this process, I've learned a lot about myself and other people. One of the things I used to tell myself was that I was a strong leader, but not the best manager. I told myself this enough times that I believed it, so I naturally avoided the managerial parts of the business and outsourced them to whoever I could. For a while, it worked, until I had an honest conversation with myself.

Sliding past the management obligations resulted in people problems. They never got better, and continual avoidance just made them worse. One day, during my weekly scheduled call with my business mentor and advisor, he convinced me that management skills could be learned, but without practice, they would never improve. And by avoiding managerial duties, there was zero chance of me improving my management skills. So I listened, I tried, and it worked. The honest conversation I had with myself was a similar one to the lesson Bedros Keuilian taught me about "the story." I had created a story about myself—that I was a strong leader but a bad manager. I bought into it. I believed it, and in doing so, I sold myself short.

I realized that the only way to become a better manager was with practice and being patient in my weakness. My skills weren't going to drastically improve overnight or even in a matter of weeks, but commitment to the skill and the learning process would produce the results I hoped for. That patience was uncomfortable, and it would've been much easier and faster to skip over it and lean into my natural leadership strengths. But that wasn't the answer. So I chose the hard right over the easy wrong.

During the process of improving my skills, I read books, talked to mentors, practiced with employees, implemented standard operating procedures, and, ultimately, slowed down. Patience requires you to be intentional with your time and presence. Being patient in my weaknesses may have felt like a step backward at the time, but in the long run, it took me many steps forward.

The Hay Is in the Barn

When you endure a process, there are going to be many parts that you enjoy and many parts that you don't. The one thing that is required, though, is a purpose behind it all. If you don't have a purpose and a reason behind the process you are about to endure, then you are never going to enjoy it, and you probably aren't going to make it. The truth is it may be a hand you're better off folding.

I would be lying if I told you that every part of every process is fun, joyful, and easy. The longer the journey, the harder it gets. But the harder it gets, the sharper we become. We should look at these long and challenging processes as blessings. They provide us with hardship, which forges resilience. They require decision-making that teaches us decisiveness. They allow us to fail, which reminds us that we aren't guaranteed or owed a successful outcome.

It's our responsibility to select goals that are built from the foundation of a personal purpose. Something that truly fulfills us. Something we want. That purpose will act as the flame that remains lit during our lowest days and toughest seasons. That flame will carry us through the process. If that flame is weak, it will go dark, and once darkness sets in, your reason to continue embracing the process will seem pointless. Easy days will feel hard, and hard days will seem impossible.

If there is one thing I'm truly passionate about it is building, documenting, and sharing the process in real time. Over the last decade, I have been able to document a variety of things. The process of building a business. The process of joining and serving in the US Army as an infantry officer. The process of prepping for marathons, triathlons, ultras, and bodybuilding shows. The process of becoming a husband and a father. My mission has been to share the processes I've experienced and learned from. Growth is not by chance; it's by choice. We have to continuously choose to remain in the fight. Otherwise, the fight moves on without us.

I love the marathon distance. It's my favorite thing to train for. It's not just about the 26.2-mile race that I complete on a given day. It's about the lead-up to race day and the process behind it. Training begins with lower volume and intensity, but as the weeks continue, the training increases. Runs become longer, faster, and harder. A prep always starts with high levels of motivation and excitement—it's the unknown that draws us in. We set big, ambitious, and intimidating goals and then fight to achieve them. At some point, however, that excitement begins to die. Fatigue begins to accumulate not only in the body, but also the mind. Mile after mile. Run after run. Week after week. This is the process that is required to successfully complete a marathon. At the peak of my prep for the California International Marathon, where I ran a personal record of two hours and thirty-nine minutes, I was running seventy-five miles each week.

After you reach the peak of a marathon build and successfully run strategically programmed workouts that tell you if you can achieve your goal or not, you begin to taper. The taper is a seven-to-ten-day period of time before the race when volume and intensity decrease. Then the work is done. At that point, it's time to shed some of that fatigue you have been carrying around for weeks to show up on race day in your greatest form. During this time, a lot of people will say, "Good luck," followed by, "The hay is in the barn."

I love that quote.

Since my dad's side of the family was all dairy farmers,

the phrase "the hay is in the barn" has always been relatable for me. It signifies a slow and steady process of putting a bale of hay in the barn one day at a time. Seeds are planted, the crop is tended to, farmers harvest, and then it is stored. You stack them up, hay bale by hay bale, until the barn is full and ready. Marathon prep is just like this. It's about all the work you've done leading up to toe the line from every workout and every training session. It's about staying focused and fueled. Healthy and recovered. All these things contribute to a successful build in a marathon prep. They all come together and are part of the process you have to endure that allows you to show up race-day ready. That is peak performance.

When I think of the process of preparing for a marathon, I picture it as an orchestra or a symphony. Back in middle school, high school, and even college, I didn't fully appreciate the synchronization that happens in an orchestra. All of these different instruments—strings and woodwinds mixed with the brass and percussion—have to come together for a singular purpose: to produce art. All these pieces are led by the conductor to produce this amazing masterpiece. I'm astonished to watch orchestras in motion because of how intense, deliberate, and focused every individual is in producing the piece. The complexity of their synchronization is overwhelming when you study it enough, but the concept is fairly simple. Each musician has an instrument and music to read. If they follow the steps on the paper in front of them, then all should unfold perfectly. But there are so many things that can go wrong from fractions of a second misplayed. To succeed, musicians must be tough. The same goes for athletes and leaders as well. We must all be tough.

To follow through with a process far enough to say, "The hay is in the barn" requires toughness. It is not an easy feat, and most people don't make it far enough in the journey to be able to say it. Most quit before the taper begins. Most lose focus on the outcome because their reason wasn't strong enough. The flame flickered too long and eventually all went dark. But when you choose to endure the process—when you can finally say the hay is in the barn, you'll know that you've stayed committed and that every obstacle you hit along the way was worth it. All the resistance was just part of the process to achieve even greater personal growth.

Forward Thinking, Backward Planning

Toward the end of 2022, I read *Traction* by Gino Wickman, founder of the Entrepreneurial Operating System (EOS). EOS is a set of concepts that has helped thousands of entrepreneurs align their organizations around vision, accountability, and results. EOS is a powerful tool when implemented into a business properly. I fell in love with the idea, approach, and methods, so my team at BPN tried it. It worked. This business model asserts that there are two distinct types of leaders in all entrepreneurial businesses: visionaries and integrators. EOS's Rocket Fuel University states, "Visionaries see the future. Integrators make it happen. These two roles could not be more different, but when they work well together, the result is what we call Rocket Fuel ... Visionaries are passionate, idea-generating, big-picture thinkers that inspire a business's success. Integrators are the steady force that transforms visions into reality." You have to know which leader you are in the business. I'm the visionary. I'm a dreamer and problem solver, and I am constantly forward thinking.

One of the greatest skills the military taught me was the concept of backward planning. I've applied backward planning to fitness goals, business goals, family goals, and even the timeline of writing this book. This concept takes a large project and breaks it down over the duration of time it takes to complete it with milestones assigned throughout. Every military operation is built on the foundation of backward planning. It begins with the objective. What is the end goal? If this plan is successful, what does the outcome look like? What is the intent? From there, you create a timeline from that day, time, and location relative to where you are right now. What needs to be done in between those two moments in order to achieve success? You create milestones, to-dos, checks, and inspections. Everything is planned, documented, rehearsed, prepared, and coordinated to ensure you stay on track.

In my experience, backward planning always increases the likelihood of success and accomplishment, but it only works if and when you are forward thinking. Forward thinking is the ability to look into the future. It is forecasting what might happen and why. It requires imagination, and while it is very much an ability, it is just as much a willingness. You must be willing to look into the future and realistically assess the possibilities. Without forward thinking, it is too late to backward plan, and your actions will follow a reactive behavior. You want to be proactive, intentional, and strategic.

A large part of enduring a process requires the ability and

willingness to look forward, into the future. Like I previously stated, if you don't forward think, you can't backward plan, and without planning, you are reacting. While reactions are normal to many different life situations and circumstances, I'd personally prefer to respond. A response, as we understand by now, is proactive, prepared, and armed for the obstacles we will experience in life's greatest journey.

Shortly after our daughter Charli turned two years old, we had our second child, Niko. At the time he was born, BPN was growing at a significantly fast rate, our team was working on some large initiatives, and my schedule was very full (in the most productive way possible). The few months before he was born were revolutionary for the business. We had just hit record-breaking sales, momentum behind the brand was electric, and we had just made a few key hires to take the business to the next level. It was an exciting time, but also intimidating because I knew my responsibilities at home were about to increase as well.

I could have waited for Niko to be born to start making a plan on how I was going to manage a growing business and a growing family, but that reaction would have set me up for failure. It would have put unnecessary pressure on my business, employees, and my wife. I knew this was not the answer, so I started planning months before our baby boy was born.

When we had Charli, I tried preparing for fatherhood as much as I could, but sometimes you don't know what you don't know. Preparation is critical, but it's not perfect. Forward thinking and backward planning can alleviate potential problems, but it doesn't guarantee your plan will go as expected. The key takeaway here is that forward thinking and backward planning will allow you to respond in a more prepared way instead of reacting emotionally. This process can reduce unnecessary stressors and issues, but you are still responsible for when the plan changes and you need to adapt.

I knew that when we went from being a family of three to a family of four that things would change. My responsibilities would change. My time would change. My priorities would need to change. So I looked into the future and started backward planning. The first step in forward thinking is identifying what you want the future to look like. I asked myself, *What does my role as the CEO of BPN look like? What does my day supporting a wife and two young kids look like?* The second step is identifying what currently holds you back or is in the way of that ideal future. The third step is to make a plan, share it, and implement it. That plan should take you from where you are today to where you want to be in the future.

If you are like me, you consider yourself a high achiever. You want to do big things in life, but you also don't want to neglect the people you care most about in the process. I knew if I didn't make a plan for my work to support the responsibilities of my growing family, I would fail. The first thing I did was make a list of key initiatives for my business. I highlighted the things that had great potential and crossed out the ones that had little to no impact on the company, brand, customer success, or culture. My team refined our focus and maximized our time by working on initiatives that generated meaningful progress. This step was eye-opening, and we realized we were working on a lot of things that were keeping us busy, but were ultimately unproductive.

Next, I reorganized our organizational structure to make sure each key initiative had an owner that was willing and able. This step came with people being promoted, demoted, hired, and unfortunately, fired. I had to ensure that if each key initiative was going to work, it couldn't directly rely on me. I delegated responsibility and empowered each individual to own the success of that project. This step required me to share my vision frequently with the most effective, clear, and simple communication methods.

Each owner of the key initiatives was responsible for the plan, and we built out teams to reach each goal. This allowed me to focus my time where I had the greatest impact on the business, on the things that I truly wanted to be working on, and show up for my family in a meaningful way for this next chapter of our lives. I couldn't have accomplished this if I didn't look forward and plan backward.

During this process, we also created an equity incentive plan for the company. I asked every full-time employee to step up and own their role. Each role was aligned with a key initiative, and I wanted them to act like owners, so we made them owners. I set aside an allocation of shares of BPN, then issued stock options to everyone on the team. It was powerful for our business and the culture. From that point on, everyone showed up to work as real owners of the company. It wasn't just my vision any longer; it was our vision. After months of forward thinking and backward planning, the changes were implemented, and I was prepared for Niko to arrive. It worked out wonderfully. It wasn't perfect (nothing is), but it allowed me to maintain momentum in the business and also show up for my family.

Be a visionary for the life you want to live and the values you want to maintain. Your ability and willingness to endure the process cannot be accomplished if you don't look forward and plan backward. Imagine what you want the future to look like. Imagine not only what you are doing, but also how you are doing it. Then make a plan, execute it, and endure every step of the way.

Run the Mile You're In

One of the most challenging parts of enduring a process, forward thinking, backward planning, and executing on that plan is remaining focused on where you are right now, in this exact moment—here. I once heard Jesse Itzler say, "Be where your feet are." If you are in the gym, be focused on the workout. If you are at dinner with your family, stop thinking about the emails you left unanswered. If you are meeting a friend for lunch to catch up, be in that conversation. Trust me, I get it, it's much easier said than done, but it's so important to be aware of our tendency to mentally jump to the next task.

As I mentioned before, this is a challenge for me during my marathon and ultra races. It is so easy to forget about the present and the mile that you're currently running because you're thinking about the next three, four, five, or ten-plus miles that are ahead of you. If you are on mile five of a marathon but you're already thinking about mile fifteen, then you are not present in the current mile. Then what happens? You lose focus. You stop thinking about your current pace, heart rate, water consumption, fueling strategy, and everything else that you are required to execute flawlessly so you can get to mile fifteen. It's very dangerous to get too far ahead of yourself. It puts your mind in a compromised position, leading you to make decisions based on where you want to be and not where you are.

Dopamine is partially to blame, but we're still responsible. I learned all about how this powerful chemical in our brains drives every decision we make from Daniel Z. Lieberman and Michael E. Long's book *The Molecule of More*. It's part of the reason we struggle to run the mile we're in—not just in reference to marathons, but life itself. Our minds are constantly battling two neurotransmitters: dopamine and the here and now molecules. Dopamine pushes us to achieve greatness, but it can also lead to our downfall. It influences us to desire something, work toward making it happen, and want more and more and more. The here and now molecules, or H&Ns, include serotonin, oxytocin, endorphins, and a class of chemicals called endocannabinoids. "To enjoy the things we have, as opposed to the things that are only possible, our brains must transition from future-oriented dopamine to present-oriented chemicals. As opposed to the pleasure of anticipation via dopamine, these chemicals give us pleasure from sensation and emotion," Lieberman and Long explained.

This doesn't mean you have a "get out of jail free card" because dopamine made you do it, but it's important to point out that there are real brain chemicals that influence us to pursue future pleasures. We have the ability to use our imagination when we look forward, and oftentimes the grass appears greener than it is now, but that's often not the case. The mile we are in has the ability to be a great one if we allow it to be.

Yes, forward thinking and backward planning involve thinking ahead to the future, but at the same time, you have to run the mile you're in. Allow yourself to anticipate this future desire that is inspired by dopamine, but don't lose focus on the here and now, or you will make decisions that can destroy your ability to get there.

I love the Adam Sandler movie *Click* for this reason. In the film, Sandler plays a character who is living a life he's not exactly happy with. He's got a wonderful wife, awesome kids, amazing parents, and a great job, but he can never find time to enjoy the present—the here and now. After meeting a strange inventor in Bed Bath & Beyond (of all places), Sandler is given a universal remote that controls time. He can fast-forward, replay, and pause life, but he doesn't have the ability to redo moments that he has fast-forwarded. Since he's been waiting for a promotion he was told was coming at work, he decides to simply skip the parts of his life he isn't enjoying so he can get to the promotion. Instead of ending up a few months ahead in the future, he fast-forwards to several years in the future, essentially skipping all these important life moments. Because he wasn't present for his family and the remote put him into "auto-pilot mode," they end up leaving him by the time he gets his promotion. When he eventually arrives at his destination, his life looks nothing like he intended or wanted.

I have never been great at running the mile I'm in when it comes to mundane life. It is a skill I'm always trying to improve. I think I've gotten better over time, but I'm by no means perfect. I'm not sure anyone is, especially those who are visionaries, set huge goals, and work to chase them down. I feel achievement through accomplishment, and it's often hard to appreciate the journey as you're in it.

Once, during one of my one-hundred-mile ultramarathons, I found myself disrespecting the race. Running one hundred miles is not easy, but the lessons learned during each race are monumental and life-changing. During this particular race, I found myself thinking about the finish line midway through the course. I stopped focusing on the mile I was in. All I could think about was mile one hundred, crossing the finish line, and being able to stop. I caught myself in this moment and will never forget the following realization I experienced:

If I'm not going to appreciate the journey, the mile I'm in, and the lessons I'm learning, then why do it at all? What's the point? For a buckle or a medal? Hell no. To keep myself focused on the journey, I've chosen to always remove the reward for the act of finishing a race; I don't keep the medals, buckles, or bibs I receive at races or competitions.

To Hold or Fold

At this point, you are probably thinking of a few processes that you have abandoned, quit, or let go. That's okay—it's normal. If you are going to commit to something for a long period of time and for the love of the journey, it better be something you are genuinely passionate about. There needs to be a meaning behind the journey, a purpose.

After talking with many successful entrepreneurs, athletes, and public figures, I have learned that there is one thing that separates them from the average person: they have chosen to explore their curiosities. We are all curious about one thing or another. It may be the business we've always wanted to start, an invention that could solve millions of people's problems, a new marketing strategy that goes against the norm, or anything else that keeps us up at night. The successful have taken action on those curiosities. Exploring these curiosities may lead to dead ends or massive victories, but you will never know unless you try. Action is the cure to most people's greatest fears and insecurities. And once you act, try, and evaluate, you can decide whether to hold or fold.

Shortly after stepping down as CEO of my business in 2023, I had the opportunity to interview Lewis Howes. At the time, I thought I was going through a mid-life crisis, but later, I found out that "crisis" was just the compounding emotional byproduct of multiple large life transitions: moving out of the CEO role in my business was the first, and becoming a dad for the first time was another. Lewis talked to me about what he called "identity foreclosure," and it has stuck with me so strongly ever since.

At that point in my life, I had been building BPN for eleven years. The business, brand, and my work had become my identity. It was all I knew, and anything outside of that was a disruption to that identity. The large life transitions of stepping down as CEO and becoming a dad had challenged all that I thought I was. Identity foreclosure doesn't necessarily mean you need to end one chapter or part of your life to begin the next. The problem that exists happens when we tie our identity to a specific job or cause and resist change.

Lewis was right. Too many people attach their identity to their job, what they do. It's okay to foreclose on that identity. Imagine a person we'll call Jack. Jack decided when he graduated high school that he wanted to be a surgeon. It was all he ever wanted to do. He got accepted into a good college to study pre-med. After graduating undergrad, he went to med school, and then completed his residency training. Twelve years later, Jack was ready to perform surgeries and make a lot of money. But now, after those twelve years, Jack didn't want to be a surgeon anymore. He didn't have the burning desire to practice medicine and didn't care how much money he could make doing it. His parents told him, "You've already put in twelve years. Don't quit now. Just put in the work for another thirty years and retire. You won't regret it!"

Thirty years! Do something you don't want to do for thirty years so you can live your last remaining years sitting by a pool, playing golf, and watching *Wheel of Fortune* until you fall asleep? Sounds horrible. In this case, it sounds like Jack should fold his cards instead of hold them. Explore your curiosities. Foreclose on the identity that you have attached to your work. Find something you are passionate about and pursue it. You are in control of your life, your work, your decisions, and the outcome. Act like it.

A year after transitioning out of the military and dedicating every waking moment to BPN, we had crossed the three-million-dollar annual revenue mark. It was just one year prior that we surpassed one million dollars in annual revenue, so the future looked promising. I heard all of these guys online talking about being a "serial entrepreneur" and owning multiple seven-figure revenue businesses. I respected these people and what they built, so I assumed it was what I should do next: start another business.

That business was called Lost Supply Apparel, and the vision for the brand was to be an outdoor apparel and accessory company. I shifted all of my focus to building Lost Supply Apparel and let off the gas with BPN. Our first couple launches with the new company went great. It was instantly generating profitable cash flow, there was a great demand for the products we were creating, and sales were very strong. During that process and all of the work to build this new brand, BPN's growth slowed down and even declined.

I had lost focus. I stopped enduring the process of building BPN, a company that was just starting to gain momentum after six years of building, and recognized I had to make a change. We closed down Lost Supply Apparel, despite the success it was experiencing, to refocus on my true passion of building BPN. Folding one process to go all in on another was one of the best decisions I have ever made. I allowed myself to explore that curiosity of starting another brand, but it didn't work out the way I intended, so I ended it just as fast as I started it.

Enduring the process requires action, but it also requires perspective. It might even require a shift in perspective. If you are going to pursue something great in life, you should expect it to come with a long and strenuous process. That process in itself is part of the reward, not just the means to an end. So if you are going to commit a lot of time and energy to something, it should be something you really care about. If it is, go all in and hold it. If it's not, then fold it. You might be doing something right now that you don't like or don't care about. If you can, fold it. End it and move on to something else. If you can't fold it, change the way you think about it. Shift your perspective because, without the right mental approach, you will never be able to endure the process long enough to see it through.

Chapter Four

CHANGE IS NOT A THREAT; IT'S AN INVITATION

"Your biggest life transition doesn't have to be a crisis or a period of loss, but rather can be an exciting adventure full of opportunities you never knew existed."
—Arthur Brooks, *From Strength to Strength*

One humid Texas night in 2022 as I sat on our back patio, I felt like my whole world flipped upside down. My life had significantly changed after two massive life transitions. We had been blessed with our first daughter, Charli Grace, and I had stepped down from the CEO role of my business. Both of these life milestones were meant to be celebrated, and they were, but something didn't feel quite right. I struggled with accepting this next chapter of my life and so much of me wanted to resist the change. I was fighting against the unknown and the newness of being a father and a founder without the CEO title any longer. The invitation to explore and embrace a new season was there, but I was holding on for dear life to the previous and familiar one.

How do I navigate building the business and being ambitious while also showing up for my family and being a good father and husband?

I felt lost, as if I was going through a quarter-life crisis. For the past decade, I had poured my heart and soul into building BPN. It had been go-go-go, from one thing to the next. Nothing had been able to slow me down, not even my mother passing away from cancer in 2019. But now I felt out of control. While the previous ten years were fast-paced and growth-focused, I felt like I always had a grasp on everything, no matter how wild and crazy things got. But now, I couldn't seem to hold on to anything. Life felt faster, days seemed shorter, and every decision I made seemed to be the wrong one. For the first time in my life, I was paralyzed by the fear of change.

When I'm positively enthusiastic about something, I tend to let everyone know. It's a contagious feeling. I want others to experience the passion, energy, and electricity behind the vision that is brewing in my mind. But when those thoughts aren't so bright, I'm not as encouraged to share. I internalize. I attempt to navigate the problems I'm feeling on my own, without asking for help—something I'm not proud of nor recommend.

On that night on my back patio, Stef came out to check on me, but I couldn't articulate what I was feeling. I tried my best to explain it to her, but it all felt insignificant compared to the problems people around me were experiencing. I was being pulled with equal power in two different life directions: drive my life's ambitions at the speed of a rocket ship or slow down enough to be actively present in the moment. So there I was, wedged in the middle, feeling like I had to choose one: be the best husband and father possible or lead BPN to its greatest potential.

There are two things I strongly believe in:

1. In order to succeed, you must be all in.
2. You must accept change to experience growth.

At the time, I was in the middle of this life transition, I truly didn't think I could manage being both the leader of my business and the leader of my family at the caliber I wanted. I couldn't see the forest for the trees. I thought I had to choose to go all in on one of them, and I thought being all in on both wasn't an option. And as someone who always preached the power of change, I felt like an imposter. I, myself, was resisting change, one that was going to facilitate the greatest growth of my entire life.

What I discovered was that my so-called quarter-life crisis was not, in fact, a crisis at all. It was just one of the life transitions we all experience. So what I came to learn, and what I will share with you in this chapter, is that change isn't a threat to our security and safety but an invitation to something bigger and potentially better. Regardless of what the transition looks like, whether it's good, bad, or ugly, it is important in guiding a powerful and meaningful life. I've learned that as much as we want to rush to find the answers during these natural life transitions, it's sometimes best to embrace the lull between chapters. Embrace change because it is not a threat, but an invitation for growth.

Let Disruption In

I have found that one of the best ways to navigate the obstacles of life is by continuing to be a student. For me, this means reading books, listening to podcasts, and having deep conversations with close friends and mentors. And sometimes the most perfect message meets you at the most perfect time of your life, when you need it most. This happened to me when I picked up *From Strength to Strength* by Arthur C. Brooks.

"Transitions feel like an abnormal disruption to life, but in fact they are a predictable and integral part of it. While each change may be novel, major life transitions happen with clocklike regularity. Life is one long string of them, in fact," Brooks said.

Life transitions are normal, and we often mistake them for a life crisis. While crises do exist, they aren't as common as we want to believe or embrace.

For years, my identity was wrapped around my work. I started the business in 2012, and for over ten years, I filled it with a lot of blood, sweat, and tears. Even though I wasn't planning to change that approach for the next twenty or thirty years, *how* I poured myself into BPN needed to change. That's because I had changed for the better.

When Charli was born, I thought I knew what being a dad would feel like, but honestly, I had no clue. It's better than I expected. It's harder than I expected, but it's also more rewarding than I expected. It changed my life in more significant ways than I expected. I'm not the same person I was before becoming a dad, and in my opinion, I'm a better man because of it.

I never expected feeling lost as I tried to figure out how my mission had evolved and how my self-identity had changed. I needed to regain clarity on those things. As someone who is naturally a doer and a fixer, I wanted to implement an overnight fix. But I realized that this was different. This wasn't like some of the problems that happen in a business. For example, when you have an employee that's not working out, there's a pretty simple fix. You can put them on a performance improvement plan, and if they don't improve, you can let them go for the best interest of them and the organization. If your company website goes down, you can reach out to your developer and work nonstop for days until it's fixed. If you're not acquiring as many customers as you were the previous month, you can implement a new marketing strategy. Those are all simple fixes and can be solved with a "block-and-tackle" type approach. As one problem arises, you identify it, tackle it, solve it, then scan for the next problem to present itself, so you can block and tackle all over again.

What I was experiencing wasn't going to be fixed overnight or instantaneously. The block-and-tackle approach didn't work in this case. These big transitions in life require a lot of deep work because life is more complicated. Life is chaotic. And while transitions can make us feel overwhelmed, the chaos doesn't necessarily need to be tended to but maybe just recognized.

Transitions are not going away. You've probably experienced them already and will definitely be faced with them again in the future. It's best to accept that so when they do happen, you are more prepared to address them. They will be distractions and obstacles if we allow them to be, but what if we viewed them as speed bumps instead? What if they were designed to be placed in the right places at the right times to slow us down? My advice: don't try and find another path around them, but instead go through them.

Okay, I thought to myself, *I'm not crumbling. I'm just trying to navigate a life transition right now. Let's take it step by step. How do I do this?*

Life transitions—life disruptions—are going to happen. It's not a matter of *if* but *when*. The question is how do you adapt and change with them? How do you use them as a strength and opportunity and not as a negative or an obstacle? How do you accept the change and adapt to thrive in it and not just survive?

We should never avoid a life-disrupting change, nor should we ever fear changing our identity. For some reason, as people get older, they tend to carry a lot of pride around the fact that they have become stubborn with age. They are less interested or likely to change their routines, habits, food preferences, and opinions. I might not be old enough yet to understand why age is often accompanied with resistance to change, but I hope that, in my later years, I don't become closed-minded. An approach that shuts down new opportunities and experiences will hold you back from reaching your greatest potential.

In the past, I have tried to fight my resistance toward life transitions by essentially "muscling" my way through them. But sometimes you just have to let them happen. You have to simply pivot, adjust, and just be a part of the transition so you can learn through it.

Think about it this way: when you're about to get into a car accident, they tell you not to tense up. You want to be as loose and limber as possible because it will mitigate the risk of injury. But if you tense up and tighten your muscles, you're probably going to sustain more injuries. So instead of trying to fight against transitions in life when they happen, try your best to truly embrace them and allow them to happen. Feel their effects and remain calm and collected throughout the process. Be patient and don't try to muscle through it.

Some transitions can actually pivot your life and put you on a whole new trajectory that helps you achieve more happiness, potential, and fulfillment. They become a blessing rather than a curse. So it's all about recognizing that. That's what I'm currently navigating in my life. My mission has evolved, and it feels clearer now than ever before.

Make Change an Intentional Choice

Have you ever heard the quote "If it ain't broke, don't fix it"? That's like asking someone how they are doing and they respond with "Fine." Not broke is not the same as thriving, and fine is not the same as great. We can be alive, or we can thrive. That experience is not based off the hand of cards we are dealt but on the choices we make.

If you are like me, you want to improve. You want to get better. You want more out of life. You want growth. Well, it doesn't happen by chance. Growth is a choice and usually an inconvenient and uncomfortable choice. Your life may not be broken—it may be fine—but is that enough for you to thrive while your heart is still beating and your mind desires more?

After Charli was born, it almost felt like my previous life died. I think I was figuring that out for a few months, and that's why the transition was so tough. I think I didn't want to let go of that previous life. But then I realized, *This new life could be better. A whole lot better.* But I had to be willing to change with it. I had to be willing to invite the new life in. I had to realize it was not a threat against the life that I had previously lived. One life does not have to die for the other to begin, but we can build off of our past to create a stronger future. I learned this lesson the hard way.

One of my favorite books is *The 15 Commitments of Conscious Leadership: A New Paradigm for Sustainable Success* by Jim Dethmer, Diana Chapman, and Kaley Klemp. In it, the authors talk about how you have to lean into your area of genius, the gifts and skills you have that can lead you, and the people around you to achieve the goals that have been established. This is what allowed me to step down from the CEO role at BPN. I truly believed my area of genius was creating emotional connections with people through content and stories. "Brand amplification and awareness" was what I called it. At the time, I didn't believe I was the right person to take the organization to the next level of growth while also trying to start and build a family. I didn't have the confidence in my ability because I convinced myself it was not my area of genius. So, I stepped down and hired a professional. I didn't believe the playbook I ran to get my company to the level it was at was the same one needed to level it up.

After hiring a CEO and shifting my focus to what I believed was my area of genius, I made the intentional choice to completely change my environment. I had to disrupt everything I knew from the last decade. I wasn't starting over, but evolving. Someone had to pioneer that charge, and I wanted it to be me. I could have easily stayed in Texas doing the same thing, talking about the same topics, and filming the same videos. But I felt part of me was starting to go into autopilot. It's almost like I fell into a coma. Complacency had sunk in, and I wasn't feeling challenged in a way that I had in the past. I needed something new. A new race wouldn't cut it. A fitness goal wasn't the answer. A new business venture wasn't of interest. I wanted to thrive again. So, I created challenge for myself and for everyone around me.

I moved my family and a small creative team to Nashville, Tennessee, a few weeks after making the decision that change was the answer. One of my greatest strengths, which can also be one of my greatest downfalls, is that I make decisions quickly, and I act on them even faster. Faster than you could even imagine. We sold our house nine hours after listing it and were on our way to Nashville to lead the charge for what I thought was the next chapter of BPN. My wife and daughter flew to Tennessee with my mother-in-law, the movers packed up our home, and I drove twelve hours north with our two dogs to our new house. Even I was surprised by how fast everything happened. But growth requires change.

We built out a new office downtown on the outskirts of the city, which was one mile away from the notorious Broadway Street that is lined with country bars and restaurants. It was noisier then our office in Texas, full of life and, to be honest, a bit uncomfortable. But growth should be uncomfortable. Change is uncomfortable and oftentimes inconvenient. You will never know the right answer for the right outcome if you never try.

———

In the 2023 documentary *Sly*, Sylvester Stallone shared his story about how he wanted to be an actor but was told by everyone that he never would be one.

"They said, 'It's just not gonna work. Maybe you'll be an extra,'" Stallone said. "So I started to buy into that. Because every time I was cast, it was always for a thug."

So Stallone decided to write parts for himself since no one else would give him one. While broke and struggling to find work, Stallone wrote the screenplay for *Rocky* and got some producers to read it. They loved it and offered him $360,000 for the script on the condition that he didn't play the role of Rocky. Stallone turned them down.

Sometimes when you have a true passion but you don't have the creative genius for it just yet, no one is going to give you the opportunity, so you have to create your own opportunity. Stallone wanted to be an actor and found a way to do it.

In the documentary, Stallone is shown living in an

absolutely stunning house on an amazing property, and the movers are coming in and packing up his stuff. He is moving to another region of the country because he has reached a point in his professional and personal life where, creatively, he is stuck. He knows that in order to facilitate growth in his life, he needs and requires change, a physical change. So he's moving out of the home that he had built for years and years to somewhere new so he can have a fresh perspective and really spark his creativity.

I needed that kind of evolution in my life. Not a revolution. No, a revolution would be if I suddenly went back to the military. I needed an evolution. Life is full of evolutions made up of small, subtle changes that build on top of each other. I used to think that everyone thought the way I thought, that everyone wanted to evolve and grow all the time. But I finally realized not everyone wants to grow, and that's okay. That's their choice. But it's not the way I think.

If I'm not evolving and growing, it doesn't matter how much money I have in my bank account. If I'm not evolving and growing, I will be unhappy and unfulfilled. It goes back to what Chadd Wright was talking about when he realized he needed to run the Cocodona 250.

"I know that if I stopped showing up—humbling myself, putting myself in these environments where I'm the new guy, where I don't know anything, where I'm going to get crushed—I might as well be dead. I'll never stop doing that."

For my family and BPN, the evolution ended up being the move to Nashville. It was an opportunity to be creatively inspired, bring new ideas to the table, innovate, and execute. It was a place where I could hyper-focus on less and produce more meaningful work. It was a change that we chose in or-der to facilitate the growth we wanted to create.

We chose Nashville for a few reasons. First, when I met Stef, she was living in Nashville, and I was living in Aus-tin. Both cities have similar characteristics but are unique in their own way. Nashville was familiar to us, but also had many new opportunities to explore. Like Austin, it embraces creativity, fitness, and an entrepreneurial spirit. Stef and I are both from the northern part of the States; I'm originally from Pennsylvania, and she is from Michigan. We missed the sea-sons and beautiful fall landscapes while living in Texas. But it wasn't necessarily the fact that we wanted to leave Texas and move to Tennessee. The move was an intentional choice to disrupt our current life. It was intended to spark innova-tion and vision. It wasn't the location that really mattered at all; it was the newness of space that we desired. We knew that new spaces, places, and faces would create growth.

In all of this, I was searching for momentum, and mo-mentum is created when action is applied to vision.

It's Going to Be Inconvenient

Right before we made the move to Nashville, my wife heard a whisper in the air one day that said, "It's going to be incon-venient." Stef had heard whispers like this in the past, and they had always come to fruition, so we took it seriously. The last time Stef had this experience was when we had spent a year trying to get pregnant with Charli. The journey became quite frustrating, but one day, Stef heard a whisper that said,

"October," and a few months later, that October, we were blessed with the news that she was pregnant. Some may call it a coincidence, but we believe in God and His plan for all of us.

As we made the move to Nashville, we were prepared to experience the normal inconveniences that accompany an out-of-state relocation. Things broke along the way, the move cost much more than we expected, our water heater went out the day we moved into our new home—the normal stuff. We thought this was what God was preparing us for. We were wrong.

The first couple months in Nashville were off to a great start. My family and I were exploring a new city, trying different restaurants, meeting people, and submerging ourselves in the community, which we thought was our new forever home. The BPN creative team that moved with us quickly got into a groove, and they were producing some of their best work. The change accomplished many of the things I had hoped for.

For the first time since I can remember, I was able to prioritize my family over work, and I was actively present during the time we spent together. I wasn't constantly checking emails or Slack or responding to text messages. The separation from the day-to-day of the business allowed me the time and space to think deeply, work "on" the business instead of "in" the business, and plan for the future rather than react to the present. I was finally able to separate my personal identity from my work, and that was something I had hoped to achieve with the move.

For those first couple months, we were in the "honeymoon

phase" of change. This is the phase where the newness creates energy, fulfillment, and motivation, but until that honeymoon phase is over, you can't accurately evaluate the results and outcomes of the change you chose to pursue.

When you commit to change and endure the process that follows, there will be many lessons learned from the experience. We can plan and plan and plan, but during that process, we will be faced with inconveniences. These are the small things that pop up when we least expect them. They can influence us to question our decisions to pursue growth and the route we have chosen. But these inconveniences are normal. They are gut checks. They guide our trajectory in the process, but also test our commitment to the journey.

Like my dad said when I first started BPN, "If it were easy, everyone would do it." Those inconveniences along the way keep us honest and humble. They are there to ensure we really want to experience the growth that is on the other side of the choices we make.

2:39

A lot happened in 2023. Along with moving my family and a small creative team from Austin to Nashville, we were in the middle of running a financial process with an investment bank to close a private equity partnership with BPN. If and when the deal was finalized, there would have been a cash injection on BPN's balance sheet, and I would have personally walked away with a significant amount of money. It would have been life-changing, and, more than that, it would have been a generational inflection point. The process started in early 2023, and we were getting very close to closing it as the year was coming to an end.

At the same time, I transitioned my training to prepare for the California International Marathon. My goal was to run a sub–2:45 race. It would be another hurdle to cross, another page in my journey, another accomplishment to achieve, but more importantly, an opportunity to prove myself right. To prove to myself that I could continue making progress, no matter life's circumstances, if I remained focused and worked hard.

Days before the marathon, I got a late-night call from the managing director of the investment bank we were working with. He informed me that the deal fell apart. It wasn't going to be moving forward. We weren't going to get it across the finish line, at least not in the near future. The way it was worded was, "Pencils down."

We had been warned. The closer you got to the finish line, the tougher things became. Nothing was official until the money was wired. Things had become more stressful, requests had become more demanding, people started showing some of their true colors, and suddenly, it was over. It was disappointing, but I honestly wasn't angry. I wasn't sad or frustrated. I knew, based on the way the deal was structured, that neither party was going to be happy with the outcome we were working toward.

Now, I believe I should give this situation a bit more context. Up until this point, since starting BPN from my college apartment in 2012, I had not taken a significant amount of money out of the business. I continued to reinvest our profits to maintain the growth and health of the organization. When I was presented with the opportunity to bring on a private equity partner, sell a minority of my shares, and take care of my family, I thought it was the right financial decision. The process of working with an investment bank and sourcing the right partner took about a year before it all fell apart. It was extremely time-consuming and a large distraction from my work and personal life. Like I mentioned, the deal started off great, but eventually, it was structured heavily against me. Before t's were crossed and i's were dotted, I knew it wasn't a good deal, but after investing so much time, money, and energy into the process, I was willing to see it through. So, when I say I wasn't disappointed, angry, sad, or frustrated when it didn't work out, I truly mean it. It wasn't the right deal, right partner, or right structure for myself and my company. It also wasn't the right time.

Since the deal fell apart just days before the California International Marathon, I went into the race with a different type of motivation and energy. I knew, without a doubt, that I was going to run a sub–2:45 marathon. Despite all the things that were going on in my head, I was in peak marathon condition, the best shape of my life. No one would have known it at the time, but the months leading up to that race were some of the most stressful of my entire life.

I crossed the finish line in under two hours and forty minutes. I was extremely happy and proud. At the end of the race, I kept telling my team how proud I was of this one. This race meant a lot to me. It was more than finishing in a certain amount of time or holding a specific pace. This performance was about resiliency. It was about staying focused and disciplined when it would have been much easier to use the last few months as an excuse.

You can take a lot away from a person, but you can't take their discipline. You can take their money, their time, and every asset they have to their name, but you can't steal their hope. Very few people knew just how difficult 2023 had proven to be for me and the team. Crossing that finish line at two hours and thirty-nine minutes felt like so much more than just a finished marathon. The preparation had paid off. The race was a reflection of all the preparation.

At that moment, my job was simple. Finish the race. Not just as a runner but as a business owner. While I was running, I heard all these people cheering, "BPN!" and, "Go One More!" And that was when I realized I wasn't just running for myself. I was running for all the people who believed in the brand. The people who woke up every day and pushed themselves. The people who wanted more out of life, who desired greatness, and who wanted to fulfill their purpose through a meaningful mission.

I didn't run the race to prove to myself I could run a sub–2:45 marathon, but to show everyone else in the world that your wildest dreams and expectations can come true. This race was for everyone at BPN. This race was to show that if I could do it—with everything going on in my life at the time—so can you.

———

A few months after moving to Nashville, the honeymoon phase had worn off. My perception of the move began to feel more uncomfortable than ever before. I missed the team back in Texas. I missed leading the organization that I spent the previous decade building. I felt guilty for abandoning the team back in Texas, who uprooted their lives to work for BPN. Some of those people left previous jobs to join me on the journey of building a brand, and others moved from out of state with their families. With each passing day, I felt worse and worse. I would cry myself to sleep thinking about what I left behind and questioning every decision I made in the previous six months. I chose growth. I experienced growth. We experienced growth. And in that experience, I learned more about myself, my family, my team, and my business than ever before.

There was only one thing left to do. Just as fast as we moved to Tennessee, we moved back to Texas. We sold our house, shut down the Nashville office, and moved the entire creative team back to BPN headquarters. I decided that if we were going to make this change, I was going all in. We made the move, and I placed myself back in the CEO role of the business.

This was the inconvenience God was telling us about. Stef and I moved our entire family and three team members to a new state for a different approach. It disrupted the business while simultaneously stimulating growth in different ways. The move was the right decision at the moment until it wasn't. The easy, wrong choice in this situation would be to think, *Well, we tried, and it didn't work, but we're here now, so let's just try and make the best of it.* That's surely one way to approach it, but not my preferred method. The hard, right decision was to think, pray, plan, and make a decisive decision before executing on it. That's what we did. We were swift and decisive. With endurance, we conquer, but with decisiveness, we survive.

You aren't always going to make the right choice, and that's okay. But you have to be willing and able to make another choice when you realize you didn't make the right one initially. Change is not a threat; it's an invitation. You can accept that invitation to pursue the journey and embrace the inconvenience that accompanies growth or you can choose complacency. You can't have your cake and eat it too in this case. You can't choose both.

By the time we decided to leave Nashville, we had been there for almost six months, and we really did think it was going to be our forever home, but things change. Life throws you a curveball sometimes, and the only thing you can do is sit back on that right leg, wait for that pitch to come in, and swing. You adapt, you pivot. That is what life is all about.

Embrace Change

Whenever I run, I either listen to a podcast or an audiobook. One of my favorite podcasts is *Founders*, where host David Senra reads from biographies and autobiographies and shares his thoughts on them. In one particular episode, Senra mentioned how everybody fears change and that change breaks the brittle.

Why does change scare so many people? Maybe it's because of their pride. Maybe it's their doubt and insecurities. Maybe it's the emotions that arise when someone's ideas or actions are challenged. Regardless of how scary change might be, if you want to be the greatest at what you do and if you want to reach your full potential, there is something that's going to have to change along the way. And if you're afraid of making that change or you don't want to confront it, you will never get better. And that weakness will surely break you.

The strongest people embrace change. They want constructive criticism. They want to become better. Amateurs constantly want to be patted on the back, praised, and told how well they are doing, but professionals want feedback. They want to know what they can be doing better and how. Professionals embrace change.

Over the years, there have been a lot of people who have worked with me and for me who have been broken by the many changes we have implemented. The strongest employees have evolved through the many struggles of working at a startup company, and many of them are still with me today. BPN has constantly been changing, evolving, and growing because we have had to in order to survive. And in a lot of ways, BPN is still considered a startup, even though I've been at it for twelve years. Working for a startup can be extremely challenging. There is constant change, and new systems are always being established. You do what you have to do to keep the business growing, developing, and thriving. This means you have to think differently and creatively. You cannot become complacent, and your foot can't come off the gas. Startups are filled with change, and if you don't embrace it, you won't survive. For many people, this type of business culture is everything they don't want in a professional career, but for others, like myself, it is exactly what I want and need.

The intent isn't to change just to change. Change still needs to be intentional. I don't wake up every morning asking myself, "What should I change today?" But with each new day, I try my best to not fight the necessary evolutions in life that provide opportunities to grow and improve. If we don't evolve over the course of a lifetime, we die. There is a reason we don't live like cavemen anymore. It wasn't an efficient or productive way to live. We have evolved as a species.

These changes don't have to be extremely disruptive to your way of life, although they may be. It might be something as small as changing the time you wake up in the morning so you can complete your workout before your kids wake up. It might be changing your diet and food choices to live a healthier lifestyle. We don't have to go out of our way looking for changes to make, but we should be willing to embrace change when the right opportunity exists.

And when change happens, don't let it break you. Change will break the brittle, but not you. Change makes the strong stronger.

Prune the Roses

One night when our BPN team was in Nashville working on some projects, we went out to dinner and I saw my pastor, Lyle Phillips of Legacy Church in Nashville, having dinner with Dr. Henry Cloud. I had just finished Dr. Cloud's book called *Trust*, so when I went over to say hi to them, I was a bit starstruck. I couldn't help but share how much Dr. Cloud's book meant to me and how it had come into my life at the perfect time. I explained how my family had moved to Nashville a few months ago and how we were already planning to move back since I decided to move back into the CEO role of my business.

"You've got to read my other book called *Necessary Endings*," Dr. Cloud told me. "It's perfect for you right now."

That night, I downloaded it on Audible and started listening to it. To this day, it's one of my favorite books. In it, Dr. Cloud talks about pruning parts of your life. But before doing that, you have to know what you are pruning for. As Cloud wrote, "You can't prune toward anything if you don't know what you want. You have to figure out what you are trying to build and then define what the pruning standards are going to be. That definition and those standards will bring you to the pruning moments, wherein you either own the vision or you don't."

There comes a time when we have to end certain things that we're doing or relationships we have in order to allow the rest of our lives to flourish. Dr. Cloud uses the example of pruning a rosebush. If you've ever owned a rosebush, you know you have to prune it by cutting away the dead roses, thorns, and stems from time to time. Those dead roses, thorns, and stems aren't helping the rosebush grow. In fact, they are holding the rosebush back from becoming healthier and stronger. When you prune the bush, it looks bare for a period of time, but eventually, it will grow back bigger and truly flourish. All of those pieces that were pruned off were actually sucking away nutrients from the parts of the bush that had more potential to grow. You have to do the same things with your life. That requires necessary endings.

"Getting to the next level always requires ending something, leaving it behind, and moving on," Dr. Cloud wrote. "Growth itself demands that we move on. Without the ability to end things, people stay stuck, never becoming who they are meant to be, never accomplishing all that their talents and abilities should afford them."

Change is necessary in life, but sometimes that change doesn't bring the results we want. Sometimes we have to make necessary endings. If there's something you know you have to do—something you have to end—you have to do your due diligence and make the most educated and responsible decision you possibly can. Sometimes you're never going to know the right or wrong answer, so you have to follow your gut with all the information you have. You have to make a decision. And sometimes that means you have to end the chapter.

That's how our move to Nashville felt. Deciding to leave Nashville and go back to Texas was one of the hardest decisions of my entire life. After disrupting the business by moving to Nashville because I thought it was the right thing to do, I realized pretty quickly that it wasn't the best decision I could have made. For a period of time, I tried to figure out how to make it work. Maybe we could slowly start to move back to Austin, or maybe we could split our time between the two cities. We could just stay in Nashville and ride things out. But I knew I needed to make that necessary ending. I had to have those hard conversations with my wife and my team.

Those were some of the hardest conversations I've ever had because I knew those decisions weren't just affecting me, but my family, my friends, my employees, and their families, too.

Change can be hard, especially after you make a choice that ends up not playing out in the way you intended. But you have to make the decision and move on from it. If you don't make the decision and prune what needs pruning, you'll end up holding yourself and others back, and you will never get where you want to be in life.

I compare the move to Nashville to playing blackjack at a casino. Is it better to play your chips or hold them? The truth is you'll never know unless you try. Let's say you get $1,000 worth of chips, then you go to the table and you sit there. If you don't play any of your chips because you're afraid to lose them, then you're simply wasting time. I wouldn't consider that strategic or smart. I would consider that being scared. You're scared to lose your chips. Not only that, but you're scared to try to win some more in the process. It's better to place the bet. Place the bet, and if you lose or fail, I guarantee you won't make the wrong bet again. I guarantee you will learn from it.

If I would have never placed the bet, I wouldn't have known if moving to Nashville was the best decision or not. I wouldn't have been able to sharpen my axe. Maybe this was a chapter in my life I needed to experience.

Do you want to get ten, twenty, thirty, or forty years down the road and ask yourself, "What if? What if I placed that bet? I wonder what would have happened?" I'm sure you don't, but you can if you're not careful. Instead, you can place the bet and learn if it's the right one or the wrong one. If it's the wrong one, you then have to make the decision to course-correct and readjust, but at least you won't be asking yourself, "What if?" decades from now.

Remember that you always have a choice. You are always in control. Don't fear change. And if it turns out that you made the wrong choice, don't be afraid to admit it and make more changes until you get it right. Those who view change as a threat will reach the end of their lives with a lot of curiosities but very few answers, and even fewer stories.

Chapter Five

IF IT MATTERS TO YOU, YOU WILL MAKE TIME

"The world is a very malleable place. If you know what you want, and you go for it with maximum energy and drive and passion, the world will often reconfigure itself around you much more quickly and easily than you would think."

—Marc Andreessen

E very day at 4:30 AM, my alarm goes off—sometimes earlier, but never later. I consider myself a morning person, so I welcome it. This is my time to think, reflect, and set the tone for the day before my family wakes up.

First, the essentials: making a cup of coffee and having an epic bowel movement. In the wise words of my good friend Matt Vincent, "You will never become number one without taking care of your number two." Next comes some mobility work and myofascial release on my lower body to prepare for my morning run. I don't typically train fasted in the morning, so I'll mix up two scoops of BPN's endurance powder, G.1.M Sport, which supplies me with forty grams of carbohydrates and seven hundred milligrams of sodium. (We created many of our products as fuel sources to improve training, recovery, and overall performance. Carbohydrates and sodium do the body wonders when it comes to endurance training.)

When I first started running, I never wore headphones, but once I became a dad, that changed. In order to maximize my time each day, I began listening to podcasts and audiobooks while I logged my morning miles. At any given time, you can find me bouncing back and forth between three to five books and a handful of podcasts. I get so much out of reading, listening, and learning from others' life lessons and experiences.

My average daily run throughout the week is between seven and ten miles. If I'm not training for a marathon or an ultra, I prefer to cover about forty-five miles each week, but if my training is more specific toward an endurance event, my weekly mileage can range between seventy-five and ninety. Just like in all areas of your life, the training and practice should reflect the outcome you desire. If the goal is a faster marathon, my weekly mileage will increase and my workouts will be highly structured. If the goal is to get bigger and stronger, my running mileage will decrease, and I increase the amount of time I spend in the gym. If the goal is to maximize the growth of the business, my workouts will be structured in a way that allows me to spend as much time on the business with the greatest energy and effort. Regardless of the goal, my training is always structured around the responsibilities of my family and never the other way around. Those decisions require intentional planning and execution.

After my morning run, I have breakfast, something quick and convenient that fuels me and tastes good. I've been eating the same breakfast for the last couple of years, and I still look forward to it every day: oats, eggs and egg whites (which I top with sea salt and hot sauce), and a banana. A few times a week, I will add wild-caught salmon or sardines to my breakfast for the additional protein and omega-3 fatty acids. And if Stef has a fresh loaf of homemade sourdough sitting out, I'll grab a slice or two in place of the oats. After that, I make breakfast for my daughter Charli and hang out with the kids. This is when Stef and I switch so she can get ready for her workout.

Even though my morning routine has evolved over the years between the demands of building the business and starting a family, there is one thing that hasn't changed: running matters.

I believe there are three things you need to start your day off right:

1. Wake up early.
2. Move your body and sweat.
3. Silence and solitude.

My "go-to" exercise is an early morning run. Running before the sun rises provides me with all three of these things. In an ever-growing, distracted world, it can be difficult to find moments of solitude, so we often have to schedule them into our routine. As a father of two young children, these moments have become even more challenging to schedule, but if it matters to you, you will make time. If you don't believe this yet, I hope you do by the time you finish this chapter.

So, why run?

It is you versus you. You keep driving through the little pieces of pain that you're experiencing in your legs. Those pieces go a long way to developing something inside of you. Your lungs burn when you first get started and you begin gasping for air as you attempt to move your legs faster than they can sustain. Running is humbling. Running teaches us discipline, focus, and the power of consistent action. Running builds confidence. And running creates opportunities for mental clarity that I haven't been able to unlock anywhere else in my entire life. It is so much more than just "running." Once you realize that, you're probably already addicted.

Running has never been natural to me. I wasn't a natural-born runner, nor did I have a natural attraction to running. I actually avoided it for as long as I could. I started running because I wanted to join the military, I forced myself to run while in the Army, and I gave it up for a short while before picking it up again. When I transitioned out of the Army in 2017, I said out loud, "I will never run a day in my life again." Well, that led to multiple marathons, triathlons and one-hundred-mile races. When I stopped running after my time in the military, I found myself missing it very badly, much sooner than I would have thought. I missed the suck, the high, the pain, and the victorious feeling of finishing a long run at the end of a hot Texas summer night. All of those feelings, the good and bad, were opportunities to grow and get better. I needed that in my life because without it, I wouldn't be able to achieve my greatest potential. I truly believe that.

I've realized there is a correlation between people who are high achievers and those who run. I'm not here to say that if you don't run you are an underachiever. I know plenty of people who kick ass in life and recoil at the thought of running. But I've met more people who kick ass in life and run. They might not even love the act of running, but the outcomes that it provides are worth the discomfort they experience.

Perhaps the simplest answer to the question of why I run is because it matters to me.

What Matters to You?

If something truly matters to you, you will make time for it. It doesn't matter what season of life you're in. You will think about it when you wake up in the morning and when you fall asleep at night. You will think about it when times get hard or when times are easy. If you don't make time for it, it's likely that it doesn't really matter to you. I've heard it many times before.

"I can't eat healthy."

"I don't have time to work out."

"I don't know where to get started."

My goal is to create an opportunity for you to have an honest conversation with yourself because I've had to be honest with myself, too. My friends, family, and mentors have called me out when I've neglected my priorities in life. I've let relationships, ideas, projects, and priorities die because I failed to "water them." Sometimes these things died because of unfocused intentions and lack of clarity, but sometimes they really didn't matter to me. And that's okay. But the honest conversation is about identifying what really matters and what you're avoiding.

If eating healthy matters to you, you will take the time to source and prepare foods that fuel your mind, body, and performance. Just like anything else that may be new to you, there is going to be a transition period. That transition period is where you learn new skills, create routines, and eventually build habits. Finding out what foods you should and should not be consuming might be overwhelming. The quantities in which you should consume them might also be intimidating. But again, if it matters to you, you will take the time to learn, research, ask questions, read, and educate yourself. Eating healthy is quite simple. Is it easy? For some, yes. For others, no. Without intentionality, you're just going to keep doing whatever is easiest, which is probably the drive-thru at your closest fast food restaurant.

"I don't have time to work out."

Taking care of our bodies is not a luxury for most. While I understand that there are people in certain parts of the world that lack the resources many of us are fortunate to have, this may not apply. I'm not ignorant of the fact that some people are literally trying to survive from one day to the next, but if you have time to binge-watch a Netflix series on the weekend, then you have time to work out. Running, lifting weights, training, sweating, breathing heavily, and putting forth effort with our God-given bodies is a standard, not an exception. Working out is a personal responsibility to ourselves and the people around us.

During a job interview, we are sometimes asked what values are most important to us. It's easy to respond with a list of things that we think might sound attractive. Some people even go to the extent of listing them in their social media bios.

"I have high levels of integrity and loyalty. And I'm hard-working and very committed."

It's easy to *say* this, but the truth comes out when we put these things into action. People often will say that they value certain things, but their daily actions don't demonstrate it. The same goes for the things we prioritize. I was once asked by a consultant what I prioritized in my life.

"Faith, family, my business, and leadership," I said, giving the answer I always gave.

"Okay, now, show me your calendar."

When I pulled it out and showed the consultant, she asked, "When do you find time for your family?"

"At night."

"So they're the last thing you think about."

"No, not exactly," I replied.

"When do you go to church?"

"I used to go," I said. "I don't know when I'm going to start going again. I don't have time right now."

I was doing what a lot of people do. We say something

matters to us, but it's not reflected or reinforced in our actions. I was saying that family was my priority, but I was still willing to work until 11PM or midnight every night and not be present with them. I came to a big realization. If you say something is a priority, look at your calendar and schedule to see if it reflects that priority.

While going through this experience, I couldn't help but think that I couldn't be the only one realizing this, so I Googled it. It's actually called the "Value-Action Gap." This phenomenon occurs when people act in a way that contradicts their values. It could be as light as saying you value taking care of your body and eating healthy but then choosing to live off pizza, fried chicken, and beer and never work out. Or it could be as heavy as saying you value integrity and loyalty, but you cheat on your spouse in secrecy. The better we become at closing that gap between our values and actions, the happier, healthier, and more successful we will be.

The question I hope you are asking yourself right now is "What matters to me?"

What matters? It may be things you don't want to do. It may be the things that scare you. But what matters might be the things you know you have to do in order to get to where you want to be. These are the things that define us. They forge our character. Martin Luther King, Jr. said it best: "The ultimate measure of a man is not where he stands in the moments of comfort and convenience, but where he stands at times of challenge and controversy."

Although we all have twenty-four hours in a day, to say that we have the same twenty-four hours is ignorant. A single mom with multiple kids doesn't have the same twenty-four hours as a kid fresh out of college with few responsibilities and a fresh start to life. But, at the end of the day, if something really does matter to you, you'll make time. This might require pruning many parts of your life so you can focus on the parts that matter. It will force you to make hard choices and step out of those moments of comfort and convenience to take on the challenge.

Whatever It Takes

The growth of Bare Performance Nutrition is an example of what happens when you make time for the things that matter. From the very beginning, making that time for BPN was one of the most challenging parts of building the business. After starting the company, a year before graduating college and commissioning into the Army as an infantry officer, I built BPN in whatever free time I had while attending the Infantry Basic Officer Leader Course, Ranger School, and Airborne School at Fort Benning. I continued building it while I was stationed at Fort Hood as a platoon leader and during nine months spent in South Korea on a training rotation. That nine-month rotation proved to be absolutely pivotal for myself, the business, the brand, and the rest of my life.

As I looked ahead knowing that my four-year active-duty contract was coming to an end when I got back from South Korea, I realized that I needed to fully commit to building the business. When I landed at Camp Casey in South Korea, BPN was making around $2,000 a month in revenue, so I knew I couldn't sustain a living off that. My goal by the time I left South Korea was to be earning $10,000 a month in revenue. So, every waking moment outside of work was spent on what mattered to me: BPN. While many of my peers were watching movies, playing video games, and socializing, I was building. All I was focused on, outside of my job in the military, was learning how to build—a business, a brand, and my future.

My dad and brother, Preston, were back in Pennsylvania managing the operations and logistics. It sounds a lot more professional than it really was. We had a spare bedroom above the garage in my parents' house, and that is where we stored inventory and packed orders. Preston had graduated from college a few months prior and was working full-time in purchasing and procurement for a restaurant supply and equipment distributor. We were bootstrapped, scrappy, and lean as could be, but our passion ran deep and strong.

A typical day in South Korea found me waking up extra early because of the time difference so I could talk to manufacturers or anyone I needed to back in the States. Then, I would spend my full day at work with the Army. Once I got off work, I would come back to my barracks room and work on BPN. I didn't know where to get started, so I began by studying the greats. I learned how to tell stories by watching Casey Neistat's YouTube videos. I learned branding by observing how direct-to-consumer companies posted on social media and rolled out advertising campaigns. I learned how to rebuild our website by migrating our e-commerce platform to Shopify and learning basic code functions. I would send handwritten thank-you notes to everyone who placed an order that week. And I documented every step along the way, filming the process as I was enduring it and sharing it with the world online.

I was all in. I was obsessed. Everything that had to do with BPN mattered.

Within ninety days of being in South Korea, BPN went from $2,000 a month in revenue to $10,000 a month in revenue. Goal accomplished. Win achieved. Confidence boosted. But in the words of Kobe Bryant after game two of the 2009 NBA finals, "What's there to be happy about? Job's not finished." I was proud, but I wasn't satisfied yet. I was just getting started, but I needed that win.

Before this story unfolds any further, I want to make it obvious what that $10,000 revenue goal meant for me. As an entrepreneur and business owner, revenue goals can be used to evaluate your performance. It is not the end-all-be-all, but it can tell a story. It very quickly paints a picture of health, growth, decline, or strategic business decisions. At this point in my journey, I needed to grow the top line or we wouldn't be in business much longer.

It would have been very easy to decide that I was going to wait until I was out of the Army to pursue building my company. But why wait? The passion was there. The energy was there. It mattered to me. Even if I didn't have the time, I would make the time. There is a fine line to straddle between being patient and striking with clear intent and purpose. We often plan our lives five, ten, fifteen, twenty years out as if we are guaranteed those years, that time, and the opportunity. But we're not. We aren't guaranteed or owed anything, but we are responsible for everything. That responsibility should act as the source of truth and North Star for every decision we make, and what we choose matters.

Before I left South Korea and made my way back to Texas, I called my brother to ask for his help. As the demands for the business increased, he was packing orders in the morning before he left for work, packing orders when he got home from work, and responding to customer service tickets late into the night. I couldn't have ever done it without him. I asked him to quit his job in Pennsylvania and move to Texas to go all in on BPN alongside me. A few days later, he quit his job and had a U-Haul packed. No questions asked. No convincing needed. Done deal. That's a partner. That's my brother.

I landed back in the States in October of 2016. That next year was absolutely wild. It was one of the hardest times of my life, and at the same time, it was one of the best times of my life. I reminisce about those days frequently. Not in a "those were the glory days" type of way, but in the sense that those were the days that laid the foundation for where BPN is today. As challenging as those years were, we were riding the high of our life. Every day was hard. We nearly ran out of money on multiple occasions. We were learning all about supply chain, inventory management, financial modeling (which we weren't any good at, but luckily, we have a CFO now), and how to operate a business that generates seven figures in revenue annually. But no matter how bad of a day we had, the amount of stress we were under, or how close we felt to losing everything, every morning felt like Christmas Day. It's that feeling when you wake up and can't get out of bed fast enough. There is an exciting unknown to what could become of the day. That feeling is pure and raw passion. It's a drug that can't be bottled up. It has to be discovered, and when you find it, time is irrelevant. Because if it matters to you, you'll make the time, and you'll do whatever it takes.

Make the Time So You Don't Have to Find the Time

There is a clear and intentional difference between making time and finding time. When we make the time to accomplish the things we need to do, there is a proactive element to those decisions. In order to make time for the things that matter, we must look into the future and backward plan. By looking forward, we can set up a timeline, eliminate things that don't really matter, and shift responsibilities so we make the time for the things that do matter. On the contrary, when we rely on finding time, we limit our ability to identify what matters and what doesn't. We can't allocate specific amounts of time based on the priority of those things, and it ends up becoming a "If we get to it, we get to it" kind of thing. Finding time is reactive. It's the leftovers from the end of the day, table scraps. That time is rarely effective or productive. Instead, we need to focus on making the time so we don't have to find it.

Every night before going to sleep, I look at my calendar for the next day. My wife and I also briefly discuss what we each have going on and how we can best support one another with work, the kids, and household chores. This is our look into the future: the next twenty-four hours. From there, we can backward plan accordingly so we can make the time for everything that needs to be done.

My nightly routine, which takes fifteen to twenty minutes, includes preparing my meals for the next day, charging any devices I may need, laying out my running clothes, and preparing my supplements. I know that from the time I wake up to the time I get to the office, which is about four and a half hours, every minute matters. Over the years, I have become more and more efficient, which has allowed me to make the time to get everything I need done before jumping in the truck and heading to BPN. In order to make the time in the morning, I prepare as much as I can the night before. Even the smallest details help. I lay out my running shorts and socks, ensuring the socks are not inside out (seconds matter). I place my running shoes by the door and untie the laces from the previous morning's miles. I mix up my fuel and put it in the fridge. All the supplements I consume right after returning from my run are laid out on the kitchen counter. I pull out the pans I'll need to cook my eggs, and I even leave a banana by the front door so I can grab it as soon as I walk back into the house. All of those things may seem excessive and that they don't actually save *that much* time, but these steps of preparation are cumulative. I do these things every day for many parts of my day, and it does make a difference. Those extra couple minutes I save allow me to answer a few emails, catch up on some work from the previous day, or even just have a few moments of silence before the kids wake up. Those minutes matter to me, so I make time for them.

While making time helps us with short-term planning and decision-making, it's also very effective with long-term accomplishments and achievement in life. When I started BPN in 2012, my life looked very different compared to what it does now. I had few responsibilities. I was single with no kids, no dogs, and no mortgage payment. I'm very happy I decided to get started when I did because I don't think I could do the same thing right now. It took all of me and all of my time to build this organization into what it has become. If I were to try and do that same thing today, I would be forced to sacrifice time and moments with the people I love, including my wife and kids. I made the time back then so I wouldn't have to try and find the time later.

If something really does matter to you, make the time now. If you don't make the time now and rely on finding the time later, it might never happen. It will always end up being the leftovers. Making the time now may feel impossible based on what else you have going on in your life, but life doesn't slow down. Life doesn't get easier, and responsibilities rarely decrease. Right now is the perfect time to start making the time because if you don't, you will catch yourself saying, "I'll find time later."

Later isn't guaranteed, but right now is.

The best way to get started is simple. Easy? You probably know the answer by now. No, it's not always easy, but the question is how much does it matter to you?

Start by identifying what actually matters to you. Next, look at your calendar. Are you making time for those things that you say matter? If not, there are clear opportunities for improvement. Now, start pruning. What can you eliminate from your days, weeks, and life altogether? There may be things you are doing, spending time on, tinkering with, or exploring that take time away from the things that do matter. Practice forward thinking and backward planning so you can build out a strategy and establish boundaries to protect your time.

You are now prepared to start making time so you don't have to find it.

Routines Versus Responsibilities

Starting a new routine, sticking with it, and turning it into a habit is personally fulfilling. It's often the result of consistency and hard choices. Normally, at some point in that evolution, there are temptations that will attempt to distract us from our goals, but with discipline, we can adapt and overcome. When all is said and done, and a healthy routine is established, it's hard to break it physically and mentally because it works. It's trustworthy. In its best form, it allows for a flow state and daily optimization. But what happens when our routines get in the way of our responsibilities? Which one do you choose?

When I was younger, I didn't understand the difference between routines and responsibilities. I assumed that a routine was a responsibility and vice versa, but I was wrong. The Law of Responsibility states that you are solely responsible for everything you have or don't have. You are responsible for everything you achieve or fail to achieve. And you are ultimately responsible for who you become. A routine can support your responsibilities, but it should not be prioritized over a responsibility on its own.

The eating disorder that took over my mind and body at fourteen years of age controlled me with great power. I was addicted to the feeling of self-control and discipline in an unhealthy and dangerous way. I was killing myself. Slowly. But that control felt so rewarding. The delayed gratification I got from ignoring hunger pangs, the temptation of food, and the audible groans of my stomach left me feeling accomplished. These rituals became routine. Working out excessively? Routine. Skipping the first two meals of the day? Routine. Going to bed hungry? Routine. It was my responsibility to take care of myself, eat food, live a full life, and socialize. Do anything but starve myself. I was so focused on the routine, the discipline, and the control that I neglected my responsibilities. My priorities were off.

Later in life, I encountered a disruption to my routine, which conflicted with my responsibilities. Before our kids were born, I would wake up at 5 AM, take my time making a cup of coffee, read a book, and respond to emails or catch up on work before heading out for a run. Sometimes I would drive to a trail, link up with some friends in downtown Austin, or explore new routes in the city. This was an essential part of my morning routine. I didn't break it for anything or anyone. After Charli was born, I assumed my routine wouldn't change much. Stef knew how much my morning routine meant to me. It was the foundation of not only my day, but my work and creativity. I viewed it as an essential part of my job. Newsflash: routines are meant to be flexible. Responsibilities aren't. I learned that it was my responsibility to be adaptable to my family's needs, not the other way around.

I didn't give up my morning routine, quit running, and embrace the "dad bod." No. I learned how to make time because it mattered to me. If that meant waking up earlier, I did. If that meant running late at night, I did. If that meant squeezing in a few miles in the morning and a few miles after work, I did. We need to show up for our responsibilities first and learn how to adapt our routines accordingly. The moment we prioritize our routines over our responsibilities is the moment we lose the trust of the people we love, care for, and work with.

Set Boundaries and Protect Them

Time is cumulative.

I heard Jesse Itzler talk about this on Joe Rogan's podcast. While discussing setting boundaries and simplifying effort toward success, Joe asked, "What was one of the first things you eliminated?" Jesse responded with, "Just saying no to the requests for my time."

Jesse went on to explain how time is cumulative. It's not just saying no to one person, one meeting over coffee, or one ten-minute sync. Those events add up and rob you of the time you could be spending on the things that really matter. Those ten-minute meetings could result in multiple missed days at the end of a year.

After moving back to Texas from our sabbatical in Tennessee, one of the first initiatives I announced as CEO was my open-door policy. I invited anyone to grab time with me throughout the day to share their concerns or ideas. It was my way of "being for the people," but that strategy quickly stole all of my productive time, and I found myself falling behind in work. The open-door policy didn't last long, and I promoted someone on our team to chief of staff to help manage human resources. I had to set boundaries so I could protect my time and productivity.

This isn't to say that you shouldn't take time to help, mentor, and support others unless it moves the needle toward your goals; however, if you continue to overextend yourself for the wants and needs of others, you will neglect your ambitions in the process. You have to be intentional with the things you say yes to and how you spend your time. You must set boundaries, but boundaries only work if they are protected, and that is a personal responsibility.

Boundaries protect your priorities. You can only sacrifice yourself, your time, or your energy for so long until you feel the effects of it. You overcommit. You don't know how to say no. You become overwhelmed and exhausted, resenting yourself and other people around you. You have to put yourself, your priorities, and your responsibilities first, or you will become useless as a contributor to society. When you board an airplane and the crew conducts their pre-flight announcements, they always tell you that in the event of an emergency, don your oxygen mask first before helping others. Why? Because if you pass out and die due to lack of oxygen, you are not saving anyone.

Am I telling you to be selfish? No. I'm encouraging you to take care of yourself so you can help other people. You will make a greater impact on the people in your life if you can show up as your best self.

Do you want your life to change overnight? (Seriously, overnight.) Then create boundaries. Protect your time, energy, and priorities. Set those boundaries, communicate them, enforce them, communicate them again, and enforce them, and communicate them again, and enforce them. This is what I learned to do in 2023. I started implementing more boundaries in my life for very obvious reasons. I found myself in a position where I was saying yes to everything and everyone. I was afraid to say no. I was afraid that saying no would come across as "I don't care" or "You don't matter enough for me to say yes." The reality is saying no is not personal. Saying no is not just for you, but also out of respect for the things or people you are saying no to. We assume, or at least I used to, that people can read our minds. We assume people know how busy we are, what we are working on, what exactly is going on in our life, and that they wouldn't ask for our time if it wasn't desperately important. But if we continue to say yes to everything, then nothing truly matters.

After Charli was born, I planned on taking two weeks completely off from work to spend time at home with our newest addition and to care for my wife alongside my mother-in-law. (Thanks, Kim. You're the best.) I didn't communicate to my team how important these two weeks were. I didn't set the appropriate boundaries. So the day after we returned from the hospital with our newborn baby, I got an emergency call from the company's leadership team. They needed me to come into the office ASAP to put out some fires we were experiencing in the marketing department. I rushed into the office as fast as I could, leaving my wife and daughter at home. One day of work turned into two days, and two days turned into three days, and before I knew it, those two weeks were spent working in the office and on my laptop at home. That was not how I planned for my first two weeks as a dad to look and feel. I was angry at my team and resentful that they stole those precious two weeks from me and my family. It took me months to realize that it wasn't the team's fault. It was my fault. I didn't set, communicate, and enforce my boundaries. If no one knows what your boundaries are, then they can't respect them. It was my responsibility, and I failed myself, my family, and my team in that instance.

I learned from that experience, and when my son was born, I took two full weeks off to spend time with my family and our newborn child. I set those boundaries early on, communicated them to the team, and they were well respected.

Setting boundaries is the first step, but communicating those boundaries and ensuring they are respected is critical for success.

Riding the Red Line

A few years ago, while I was on a plane traveling for work, I began flipping through the movie options and decided to watch *Ford v Ferrari*. It's an amazing film, but besides being entertaining, the film also taught me a great lesson. I watched Christian Bale push the Ford GT40 to its extreme limits. He would drive that vehicle so aggressively, but at the same time in the most respectful way imaginable. The goal was to get the most out of the vehicle. To take it to its upper limit. To push it to the verge of breaking down and imploding. That is maximum capacity, maximum output, maximum performance. Bale would monitor the RPMs on the dashboard, which measure how many times the engine's crankshaft makes one full rotation every minute. He would redline the GT40, which is the maximum speed that an engine is designed to handle without causing damage to the internal components of the car. If he pushed the car too hard and over the red line, he could destroy it. If he drove it too far below the red line, he would underperform and lose to his competition. The goal was to ride that red line.

Throughout the course of our lives, different things are going to matter more than others during different seasons, chapters, and transitions. What mattered to me when I was in my early twenties is much different than what mattered in my late twenties and what matters to me now in my thirties. As new priorities arise and shift, we must evaluate what stays and what goes. It's impossible to keep stacking things that matter on top of one another without reducing the focus on others. We don't have the time, energy, resources, or capacity to do it all. Trust me, I wish I did. My goal is to ride the red line, maximize my time, maximize my output, and do more while working on less. There are a few different ways you can ride that red line in life—few concepts, but many methods. I've tried a few, so I'll share with you what has worked and what hasn't.

First off, you can burn the candle from both ends. You can say yes to everyone and everything, stack as much as possible on your plate, half-ass the few things you actually get done, and hold on to a to-do list that gets longer and longer with each additional week. I lived this approach for years. I thought this was the only way to do it, but I also carried a lot of "pride" in burning myself out. This wasn't optimal or very productive. It felt like I was in a room, alone, filled with water. Slowly, the water in that room was increasing, and I was floating toward the ceiling, getting ready to hold my breath as the water flowed over my head and filled every inch of the room, including my lungs. With each additional day, I took on more responsibilities, picked up the slack from others, opted out of having the hard conversations, and volunteered myself to do more. I was riding the red line for sure in this case. I was at maximum speed, but I was far from maximum performance.

In February of 2024, when I decided to put myself back in the CEO position of BPN, I committed to doing things differently. One of the reasons I stepped back from the role thirteen months prior was because I didn't know how to ride the red line properly. I thought the only way to do it was by accepting the unavoidable collateral damage. That damage came at the expense of my family, my relationships, and my health.

During those thirteen months that I wasn't the CEO, I learned a lot. I grew a lot. I lost a lot of money, opportunities, trust, friendships, and business momentum, but the clarity I gained made up for all of it. Letting Stef know that I planned on moving back into the CEO role was not an easy conversation. She knew that the decision would require us to move back to Texas, but she was more concerned that I was going to drive myself back to burnout. Exhaustion. Zombie mode. I made a commitment that it would be different. That I would change my methods. That I would maximize performance, not speed.

After I joined the Army and finished my training as an infantry officer, I was placed at Fort Hood, Texas, with the 2-12 Calvary Regiment, 1st Armored Brigade Combat Team, 1st Cavalry Division. I arrived to my unit and was assigned to Bravo Company to take over as the platoon leader of 1st Platoon. The first thing I was told by experienced leaders, officers, and NCOs (noncommissioned officers) was to observe. Don't come in and make changes day one. Watch the platoon, learn from them, and let them welcome you to their high-functioning organization. So that is what I did. And I decided to take that same approach with BPN when I returned to the role of CEO.

The first thing I did upon my return was study the company. I had to understand what was working and what wasn't. Where we were spending our time. How we were operating. Who needed to stay and who needed to go. It was time for a change. There is a cost to change, and that cost is an investment into a future outcome, for better or worse. Like any good investor, you better place your bets wisely, conduct your due diligence, mitigate risk, and believe in the mission and people of where you are placing that money. I expressed my concerns with the BPN team, but also presented the opportunities that I recognized. My number one concern was that we were focused on too many things. We bit off more than we could chew, and now we were playing defense as opposed to offense. Every day felt like we were playing catch up, with little intention behind the purpose of our work and how it fit into the greater mission. There were endless projects we were working on that didn't move the needle for the business. We over-hired, which resulted in an unhealthy amount of overhead, unproductive employees, and a distracted work environment. We overcomplicated the business, added procedures for everything, and onboarded a different layer of software for the smallest of day-to-day operations. We even had a software that managed all of our other software. Change was not just an option; it was required.

Again, the goal was to maximize performance, and in order to do so, we had to make sure we were spending our time working on things that mattered. So, we started over. We rebuilt the organizational structure, which came with promotions, demotions, and unfortunately, layoffs, the first ones we had ever done. We turned off everything that wasn't working to test its incremental impact on the business. We evaluated where we were spending time and the return on how it was spent. We discontinued products that were underperforming and were a distraction to our marketing team. We outsourced more, removed layers of management, encouraged more "doers," and eliminated unnecessary meetings.

After all was said and done, our team was ten employees smaller, we had five key initiatives for the business, and we reduced overhead by seven figures on a twelve-month, forward-looking basis. This was not easy, and it came with a lot of hard decisions and tough conversations, but it was the only way to improve the business. BPN was doing more by focusing on less. We were riding the red line of performance in the most effective and efficient way possible.

Dealing with Unexpected Challenges

One of the greatest characteristics and strengths you can build is your ability to deal with unexpected challenges and become resilient. I've mentioned the importance of choosing to do difficult things and how they forge growth, adaptability, and resiliency. Difficult things are essential for self-improvement and development. But normally when we think of hard things, they are something we have chosen to do. This could be training for a race, setting a weight loss goal, or starting a business. All of these things require us to endure the process, but we have entered that process knowing and willing. We are able to set expectations, plan for the suck, and mentally prepare for hardship. Don't get me wrong, choosing to do hard things is essential in life and the benefits are significant, but there is something I want to address that I believe is almost more important. How do we react and adapt to overcoming hard things that we haven't chosen? What happens when we are put in a position that we didn't prepare for? Are we just as strong or does our true, authentic character break through and expose our weaknesses? We must be able to adapt to the hard things we get thrown into and that require us to be resilient—the unexpected challenges.

The US Army Ranger School was an experience that provided equal parts of hard things I chose to endure and hard things that I unwillingly had to embrace. Volunteering and training for Ranger School was a huge undertaking. This sixty-one-day tactical leadership evaluation course was designed to push you beyond your physical limits, break you down, starve you, deprive you of sleep, and demand your greatest performance despite everything involved. I failed two phases before graduating from the course, so I spent a total of 145 days there. It was the hardest four and a half months of my life, and for many days, it felt like I was never going to make it out. Ranger School started to feel like my new life. No sleep, little food, lots of rucking, and constant fear of the instructors. I learned a lot during this time, not only about myself and my potential, but also about other people. I watched the hardest and toughest men become weak and selfish. I witnessed people fight over food, saw arguments get stirred up by who was carrying more weight, and watched grown men cry when they were told they had to recycle a phase. It was challenging. It was hard. We knew it was going to be hard when we signed up. But there were things we experienced that we weren't prepared for. Things that we didn't "sign up" for.

The truth is it is much easier to choose a challenge when you know exactly what you are getting yourself into. It's easier to embrace the suck when you know what the suck entails, how long it's going to last, and what level of effort you are required to give. Doing hard things is much more difficult when you enter the unknown or when things happen that you didn't plan for or expect. We knew Ranger School was going to be hard, but a lot of guys didn't expect to be as hungry as they became. They didn't expect to do crazy things for food, like sneak into other team members' rucksacks at night and steal their MREs (meals ready to eat). If that happened to you, you could say goodbye to tomorrow's food. One of the

Army's values is selfless service and integrity. For many, it holds true, but when things get unexpectedly hard, people's true character shines through.

My time in the military was pivotal to my personal achievements, entrepreneurial accomplishments, and the man I have become today. I learned a lot about a lot from a lot of different people, including NCOs, soldiers, men, women, good leaders, and bad leaders. They all provided me with insight into what to do and what not to do. The military also forced me to learn the skills I needed to cope with the unexpected. I remember many Friday afternoons getting ready to leave work for the weekend just to be stopped by our First Sergeant. Before we could be released for the weekend, he would have to inspect the motor pool, which housed our vehicles and special equipment. If he didn't feel like leaving that night, he would find any reason to keep us there.

"Oh, look what we have here. A cigarette butt sitting here behind this vehicle. Now what we are going to do is clean the entire motor pool until it is spotless," he would say.

Five hours later, we would finally be released. Those were character-defining moments. They taught me how to deal with the suck when I least expected it. They showed me how to be adaptable, resilient, and patient in moments when I'm not in control. Our true character and values are tested when we are faced with uncomfortable environments that we didn't plan for. It's not what we do in the moments of planned adversity, but in the moments that are unplanned and unprepared.

The takeaway here is to become resilient. When hard and uncomfortable times arise, view that as an opportunity to maintain your posture. Don't allow the adversity to break your character so you can walk away from that situation with pride. Like I've said, it's much easier to combat hard things when you are prepared for the situation. How do you react when you're not? What will people say about you when things get hard? Are you the person who breaks into someone else's rucksack and steals their food? Do you become selfish and weak? Or do you lead from the front, stay true to your character, and be strong?

Exposure to unknown and unexpected hard moments provides you with the opportunity to grow and develop those necessary coping skills. You become more dependable to yourself and other people around you. You become a rock, the foundation for resiliency. You become a trusted component of the team, group, and society. Put yourself in scenarios where you have to adapt or where you don't have a plan. I promise you'll learn a lot about yourself.

Courage Is Required

Shortly after arriving in Nashville, I started focusing on my relationship with God and building my faith. I didn't want to just be a believer. I wanted to be an obedient follower of Christ. I knew a lot of "believers," and some of them suffered from the Value-Action Gap. That decision and commitment shaped the content I was consuming—the books I read, the podcasts I listened to, and the messages and people that resonated with me. Erwin McManus was one of those people.

As a result, I came across this wonderful guidance

from one of Erwin's podcasts: "I think winning is a wonderful outcome. It's just not a great purpose. Your purpose for life should be rooted in who you are. So, if your purpose is who you are becoming, it can't be shaken by wins or losses, failure or success. You should want to win. You should want to be the best. These are great aspirations. But they should be outcomes of the person that you are committed to becoming."

That statement made me question what mattered to me, and I hope it does the same for you, too. Do you want to win in life just so you can stand on the podium, raise the trophy over your head, and receive praise from people who may not remember your name tomorrow? Maybe so, but that's not what matters to me. I want to be proud of my purpose. I want to be committed to my work. I want to build the best, not necessarily the biggest. That is what matters to me, so I'm going to make time for the areas of my life that matter most.

All of these ideas are great. They sound amazing on paper and would probably make for a beautiful Instagram caption or keynote speaking event, so feel free to use them for your own material. Ideas make for great dinner conversation, and they are a great icebreaker when getting to know someone, but they don't actually move the needle for your life. The only thing that moves the needle is action. Action is scary. It's a commitment to the ideas you are so passionate about. Action requires courage, and without courage, you will never reach your full potential. Your life will end with wasted ability. And there is nothing worse than spending your time on things that don't actually matter to you. If you are spending your days, time, and energy on pursuing a life for recognition and respect from others, stop. Have the courage to take the time to understand what matters to you. YOU. Then, *make* time for it.

Chapter Six

BE ALL IN, NOT ALL CONSUMED

"I've failed over and over and over again in my life, and that is why I succeed."

—Michael Jordan

'm not against being obsessed. I'm actually a proponent of it. It's how I've built my business from nothing and how I've shaved ninety minutes off my marathon time. We need a healthy obsession to get better. If you show me someone who has reached success, I guarantee you there is a fire-burning obsession within them. Ever since my first YouTube video in 2014, I've documented my healthy and unhealthy obsessions. These obsessions have helped me achieve massive goals, push myself beyond what I once thought was impossible, and turn visions into realities. But I would be ignorant to say that obsessions don't come with consequences or sacrifices. There is collateral damage to pursuing an obsession. Some damage is expected and calculated, while others may be a surprise. Pursuing greatness comes at a cost, and only you can decide if that cost is worth it in the end. I haven't executed my life up until this point without flaws, and I don't expect to avoid mistakes in the future. But I'm aware of the consequences that come with my decisions.

A healthy obsession requires focus, ownership, commitment, and discipline. It keeps you going on the days you want to, but more importantly on the days you don't. It's what makes you self-powered. But obsession can quickly take over your life and everything around it. It can consume you in a way that causes you to neglect your family and other responsibilities. This is how food and fitness have controlled much of my life since the start of my eating disorder at fourteen years old. There are healthy obsessions that fuel your life and add meaning and purpose behind everything you choose to do or not do. But there are also unhealthy obsessions that steal your life away from you.

My running coach, Jeff Cunningham, explains obsession like this: "There is a difference between being all in and all consumed. All consumed is when we turn something into our identity, and without it, we become soulless and rudderless. All in means you compartmentalize your energy in a way that allows you to be hyper-focused on a goal without it being destructive to your professional life, your relationships, or your personal health."

There is a fine line between all in (a healthy obsession) and all consumed (an unhealthy obsession). It's easy for that line to become blurry and disappear, but having the knowledge of what each looks and feels like can help you navigate goals in a healthy way. When self-awareness meets all in, the result is powerful. On the contrary, lack of self-awareness and being all consumed is a recipe for disaster and destruction. Oftentimes you don't even realize you're all consumed until you're in the thick of it—drowning in the headspace, ignoring personal responsibilities, and lighting a fire of collateral damage behind you. The key word that I took away from Jeff's comment is "destructive." Being all consumed can, and likely will, lead to a destructive life.

I've tried to build my business in the healthiest way possible, and I believe I've done a pretty good job at it, but don't get me wrong, it's led to an "unbalanced" life with heavier seasons than others. That is the entrepreneurial journey. The key difference between a healthy and unhealthy obsession is self-awareness.

I believe self-awareness is an essential characteristic to gain clarity about your life, where it currently stands and the future you imagine. Internal self-awareness represents how clearly we see our own values and how our actions reflect those values. If you lack self-awareness right now, it's okay; you probably don't even know it. But the goal of this book is to highlight perspectives that inspire the clarity required to see your life in a new way and Go One More.

When Stef and I were getting married, we went to premarital counseling and discovered that a lot of issues we were experiencing in our relationship were because I was a workaholic. From the beginning, I was all in on BPN (and still am to this day). I believe I was born to do the work I am doing. It truly fulfills me. And I was proud of my work-work-work ethic. Start the day early and work until you close your eyes as you lay down in bed. Work 'til you die. Rest when you're dead. But I came to realize there's collateral damage that comes with that mindset. One day, while at the premarital counseling session, the therapist asked me a poignant question.

"Nick, who are you without your business? Who is Nick Bare without work?"

I was instantly offended. I thought, *How dare you ask me that.* The question stuck with me and was a thorn in my side for a long period of time. The question made me feel human-less. It was almost as if I, Nick, wasn't viewed as a person with thoughts, feelings, and emotions, but as a product or brand. I also took it as a personal attack that questioned my commitment to my wife, our relationship, and our soon-to-be marriage. But eventually, I understood this to be a great question. I've truly identified myself and everything I am with building BPN for a decade now. After investing so much into it, how could I *not* identify with what I'd built? I can understand how being an entrepreneur means you almost lose a part of yourself in the process. You sell part of your mind, body, and spirit to the business. This is when, as Jeff Cunningham said, you become all consumed.

As I've continued to grow, I reflect back on that premarital session and it brings me back to my mission in life. When I dove into starting BPN, my mission was to build it, to be all in, to be obsessed, to work. But my mission and purpose in life—my guiding North Star—has changed a lot since then.

Building BPN is still a large part of my mission, but it's not my only mission any longer.

Having a defined guiding North Star will help you navigate between being all in and all consumed. That North Star allows you to focus on the vision in front of you instead of just where your feet are in the current moment. That's the balance that requires necessary forward thinking and backward planning. It's not easy to be present in the moment and simultaneously absolutely ambitious for the future. But the more all in you can be and the less all consumed you are, the easier it becomes.

Turn Your Weakness into a Strength

Most of the time, the only thing holding us back from achieving greatness is ourselves. This is an understanding I have come to discover through lots of hardships and letdowns.

The powerful mission of Go One More was founded on failure. It began when I was about to give up on my marathon training run in 2018, as detailed in the opening pages of this book. I was choosing to quit. It was a conscious decision that I was aware of, regardless of the consequences I knew accompanied that choice. I was giving up and letting weakness win, but I ultimately chose to overcome that weakness and kept running. One foot in front of the other, over and over and over again. Those steps are the journey toward greatness, no matter how you define it. You can't get there without those first few steps.

I find it extremely fascinating that we place so much effort and focus on highlighting our strengths while neglecting our weaknesses. As I think about all my personal strengths, and maybe you could do the same, I realize that many have developed from what was once a weakness. Our greatest strengths, skills, attributes, and abilities were likely not always as well defined as they are today. The reality is no one wants to brag or boast about their subpar abilities, usually out of insecurity. But those weaknesses are opportunities. As I mentioned earlier, I starved myself as a teenager. An eating disorder took control of my mind and body. I was all consumed by food and fighting the temptation to eat due to a fear of gaining weight and accumulating body fat. Some people may find it offensive for me to consider my eating disorder as a weakness, but that's the way I see it. It definitely wasn't a strength. My mind was weak, and sometimes it still is when it comes to maintaining a healthy relationship with food, but I eventually turned that weakness into a strength because I was able to identify it as an opportunity for growth. Turn your weakness into a strength, or you'll end up letting it consume you for the rest of your life.

After the doctors identified my eating disorder, I fought to have a better diet, but for years, I struggled to maintain a healthy relationship with food. I've been criticized by talking about "relationships with food" and have been told that relationships are only built between people. I disagree, and anyone who has struggled with disordered eating will likely disagree as well. An eating disorder is like a deep cut. It heals, but it leaves a scar as a reminder. It is not something you ever completely overcome or get rid of. It is still part of me today, but I'm more in control now, and I understand the importance of fuel, food, and nutrition for a healthy mind and body. My eating disorder created an opportunity in the most positive way possible; it sparked my interest in nutrition, training, fitness, and increased performance.

I was once obsessed with starving myself, but I learned to turn that obsession into something positive. The control and discipline I achieved and refined to refrain from eating for long periods of time was powerful. It's not something I'm proud of, but it's the truth. I could go days without eating. You could've put a cheeseburger in front of me, and not a bone in my body would have inched toward it. But as my mindset evolved and I became aware of the damage I was causing myself, I learned to shift the restraint and control I developed when struggling with an eating disorder into an ability to be extremely disciplined with my wants, thoughts, and temptations. I took a weakness and turned it into a strength.

In order to get healthier, I started going to the gym. After months of breaking my body down, it was time to start building it back up. I began eating more. I made smarter food choices and prioritized my protein intake. As my body started to get stronger, so did my mind. I slowly regained confidence in myself, what I was doing, and who I was. I'm not going to sit here and tell you that it was an easy road to recovery and that all these decisions happened without slip-ups and hard times, but I committed to getting healthier. I turned my obsessive tendencies toward feeling better— not just for myself, but for my family, too. The decision to improve my relationship with food was made to achieve a specific outcome, but in the process, I fell in love with the journey. I discovered my greatest passion and life's work—an interest in nutrition and fitness—through a weakness that had the potential to kill me. And if I didn't make the choice to get better, it eventually would have.

When I applied to college, I decided I wanted to pursue a career in nutrition. Consuming food was once something I struggled with. It was a weakness. But I now wanted to turn that weakness into a greater strength so I could help others who were experiencing something similar. I knew I couldn't have been the only person who had an unhealthy relationship with food, and it was an opportunity for me to save others. While studying nutrition at the Indiana University of Pennsylvania near Pittsburgh, I fell in love with the supplement industry, science, bodybuilding, powerlifting, and spending as much time as possible in the gym. At the time, the dietary supplement industry was like the Wild West. Products were being pulled off the shelves because of banned substances. People were getting injured and landing in the hospital. New companies were launching daily and closing just as fast. It was hard to tell who was doing it right and who was just trying to make a buck. So I decided to make my own products. I started buying ingredients in bulk from reputable suppliers online and mixing up my own supplements in my dorm room.

Picture this: A food scale on my desk. All these white powders—the raw ingredients—on the counters. I would weigh my materials, blend my product, package it in clear plastic baggies, and save it for later. Once my friends and friends-of-friends started finding out what I was doing, they wanted to try it. Every day, people would knock on my dorm room door, I would hand them a clear baggie with white powder, and they would hand me a few dollars in exchange. I promise I wasn't selling drugs, but I was in the market of pre-workout. What started as a passion and hobby turned into another opportunity.

Between my junior and senior years of college, the military-associated bank USAA allowed Army ROTC cadets like me to take out a loan of up to $25,000, with a low interest rate and extended payback periods. They knew we were about to be active-duty officers with a steady paycheck and no time to spend it. A lot of my friends and peers were picking up this money and buying engagement rings, new cars, and vacations, but I saw this as my golden ticket to start my business. To be approved for this loan, we had to have the "use of funds" approved by our battalion commander, who was a lieutenant colonel. He made me create a business plan and present my idea to him. (I would love to find that original business plan. I can only imagine what I put in there and where I expected to be by this stage of my personal and professional career.) To my surprise, he approved a $20,000 loan.

The rest, as they say, is history. I found a manufacturer in California and placed a production order for "Flight," which to this day is our flagship pre-workout product. We launched with the same formula I was selling in my dorm room to all the pre-workout junkies. The foundation of the product has been maintained, but the formula has evolved over the years.

I spent all the money I had to place an order for the minimum order requirements from the manufacturer—all $20,000 on inventory. Most of the product was stored at my parents' home, which was about three hours away from my university. I stuffed my college apartment with as much as it could hold and even stored some in my car as I transferred boxes between the locations. I wish I could say it was all blue skies and rainbows from there, but that's the furthest thing from the truth. Building a business isn't easy, which is no surprise, but if I knew then what I know now, I don't know if I would have ever started. This journey has been the hardest thing I've ever done, but I would do it again and again and again if I had the opportunity. I had taken my eating disorder and turned it into something positive. I was all in with Bare Performance Nutrition.

A Meaningful Mission

As human beings in the twenty-first century, we are often highly influenced, choosing careers, lifestyles, and personal goals based on what everyone else is telling us. After conducting dozens of interviews and conversations with very successful entrepreneurs, athletes, and professionals, I've learned that these people chose a different path. Their journey is guided by a North Star—a purpose—shaped through personal ambition, desire, passion, and a meaningful mission.

The first step in proving yourself right is honestly identifying the what, where, and how of the objective you're trying to prove. What is your purpose? What does success look like for you? What do fulfillment and happiness feel like? If you don't know right now, that's okay, but these are personal questions YOU need to answer. They shouldn't be persuaded by external validation or the wants and needs of others. Without a North Star, everything will feel meaningless, and your ability to maintain your commitment will be challenged.

Without an established vision, there is no direction. A quote that guides this thought is the first part of Psalm 29:18: "Where there is no vision, the people perish." We have to put our North Star at the forefront of our lives—our relationships, our business, everything. An effective vision answers questions such as:

- Where are we headed?
- What does the path forward look like?
- What do I need to focus on right now to get there?

I love how *New York Times* bestselling author Lewis Howes defines purpose in his book, *The Greatness Mindset: Unlock the Power of Your Mind and Live Your Best Life Today*. He calls it a "Meaningful Mission." It is our North Star, our vision for where we're going. It is necessary to implement forward thinking and backward planning. And it must be intentional.

In *The Greatness Mindset*, Howes said, "When we decide who we want to become—our definition of greatness, our Meaningful Mission—then that becomes our identity. And when our identity is clear, then our behaviors are easier to establish."

Howes says the first step to discovering your meaningful

mission is to be honest with yourself about yourself. When I spoke to Howes on my podcast, he shared the following about the concept of having a meaningful mission:

"I think the enemy of greatness is a lack of a meaningful mission. . . If we're clear on the mission, then we can start saying yes and no to things that either serve or don't serve the mission. And I think that allows us to take our power and our energy back and be more effective."

Our meaningful mission provides the clarity we need to Go One More. He stated that a person without a mission has the potential to be destructive or dangerous because they're just wandering around without direction, turning in circles and going nowhere.

I'll be honest with you, I greatly dislike (my mom didn't like when I used the word "hate") when people ask, "What is your purpose?" Up until this point in the book, I have mentioned and referenced purpose many times, but I have struggled with that term for most of my life, and I want to clarify how I perceive my purpose and how it differs from my meaningful mission.

"What is your purpose?"

When people used to ask me this, I would begin to sweat. I thought I needed to have an answer that was elaborate and profound, something like "I want to change the world." But the truth is I didn't know what my purpose was. I thought my meaningful mission and my purpose were the same thing. I've learned that your meaningful mission can change and evolve, but your life's purpose is much larger than that. Our meaningful mission is something we are focused on in pursuit of achievement, growth, change, or impact. My meaningful mission in life is my work; it's BPN. My purpose, on the other hand, is to be more like Christ. It is to be a follower of Jesus and to live a worldly life that allows me to have eternal life. It is the foundation of my values, how I raise and support my family, how I treat others, and how I approach my work. My purpose is to neglect what society tells me is normal or accepted and be transformative in my walk with the Lord.

To be honest, I fought against that purpose for a long time. It didn't serve me, and I don't like to admit it, but it felt too lofty. It took me a long time to accept Jesus as my Lord and Savior, but once I did, it provided a lot of necessary clarity for every other aspect of my life.

While my life's purpose is to be more Christlike, the "purpose" behind a specific goal, event, or milestone is the why that fuels the work; it's the passion. Passionless work is unsustainable and unfulfilling. It makes it hard to endure the process. The purpose of pushing my body to its physical limits in preparation for some of these races and competitions is to maximize human potential. I'm genuinely curious about what I can achieve and how much better I can become when I commit to a process and the work that is required. I don't just do it for me, but to help others improve as well. I'm just as passionate about documenting and sharing the journey as I am about enduring it. My purpose behind a lot of my work is to instill the confidence in others that lets them know they have control of the variables in their life, and it's up to them to own that responsibility.

"If you hold a clear image of your ideal self as your North Star, you will make incremental life changes that will bring you closer to the meaningful success that you find fulfilling," Lewis Howes said in *The Greatness Mindset.*

You have a choice to live out and fulfill your purpose through your meaningful mission. When your purpose and meaningful mission are clear, you then can be all in. But when that purpose and meaningful mission is unclear, you will default to being all consumed. You will be consumed by things that don't matter, people's opinions that don't matter, and goals that, in the grand scheme of life, don't matter, either.

Knowing When to Sprint

Now, I'm usually more of a marathon guy, but I do love a good sprint every so often, especially when it comes to my work. A sprint refers to a predefined span of time in which a team or individual works to accomplish specific goals with increased intensity. I've used the sprint technique for more than a decade (even before I knew what a sprint was), and it has worked wonders. This predefined span of time allows you to hyper-focus on a task, operate with full efficiency, and achieve significant progress. These are very productive periods of time that allow you to really go all in. Sometimes you complete the goal, oftentimes you put a dent in it, and usually you are just chipping away at something much larger. The time in between sprints comes with more rest, slower operating intensity, and more planning.

I was first introduced to sprint planning when the BPN team started working with agencies in the tech space. For the first couple years of the business, I managed our website on my own until I was in over my head—way over my head. We eventually hired an agency that came with a full team, including designers, developers, researchers, and a project manager. It taught me a lot about effective product planning, development, and execution. Before this, a "sprint" to me was an all-out, full-effort movement that lasted for a short period of time until you reached physical (or mental) failure. I now like to operate my life, business, fitness, and personal goals with a sprint planning approach. These sprints differ from the normal course of your day-to-day because they require specificity, which creates powerful outcomes. The two words I want to highlight when we think of sprint planning are specificity and intensity.

The difference between a sprint and daily work activities is like the difference between working out and training. I didn't always know the difference between regular workouts and training, but when I learned that they weren't the same thing, it shifted my perspective. I no longer say, "I'm going to work out" when I head to the gym. I say, "I'm going to train." Working out is recreational. It's moving your body to promote health and wellness, but it lacks specificity. Training is specific. It requires a plan, structure, and periodization. The difference between working out and training is the specificity that is applied. Training is intentionally designed and executed. Working out is less structured and more flexible. When you go all in on something, you must show up with the training mentality over the workout approach.

Now, like I learned by working with some of the agencies that BPN has contracted over the years, sprints are pre-planned, time is allocated, and the focus is very clear. This is a proactive approach to the sprint model. It works, and in my experience, it works very well. It provides you with the time, space, resources, and intentionality to get some really strong work done. But sometimes a sprint is reactive. There is no better way to say it: you just have to get shit done. Plans change, things break, and people quit.

Sprints that are initiated by a reactive trigger will often feel chaotic, unorganized, and unsustainable because they normally are. But here is what I like to do: stop, drop, and take inventory. This isn't something I was always good at, but when you are stuck with enough "oh crap" moments, you tend to become more adaptable to obstacles. This is resiliency. We become more adaptable to a stimulus with more exposure and at more frequent intervals. So, when things keep going wrong in your life, part of you should be grateful because it is building resiliency. And resiliency has the opportunity to help you turn a weakness into a strength.

Imagine you are going through your day, blocking and tackling tasks, and you are already operating near redline when something goes wrong, and your entire world feels like it was flipped upside down. Chaos, madness, and extreme feelings of overwhelm sink in. I used to crumble in these moments, but with enough repetition, my resiliency muscle has grown stronger. So, now I use the stop, drop, and take inventory approach.

First, stop what you're doing. It's very easy to feel the need to move even faster, do more, and rush to the finish line, but you are almost guaranteed to break more things in the process and overlook productive solutions. Next, drop what you're working on. What you were working toward in that moment may not be a priority any longer because of the changes you were just hit with. Third, take inventory, not mentally but physically. Write it down. It's time to sprint. This sprint is a hyper-focused, all-in mission. Ask yourself:

- What happened?
- What does success look like if this sprint addresses the problem?
- What needs to be done (listed out in order of priority)?
- What can I do right now?
- What can I not do right now?

Those last two questions are the most important, and they have helped me alleviate stress and feelings of overwhelm and create order from chaos. Why? Although we may feel like there is so much to get done in such a short amount of time, there may be only a few things we can realistically do right now. We often stress over things that we physically can't get to for days, weeks, or even months. And many times the objectives we need to accomplish are condition-based, meaning they can only be done when a previous task is completed. From what I've found, there is much less we can actually do than we think we need to do. These feelings of stress and chaos are actually more self-induced problems than external issues we are dealing with.

Lastly, take action. Action eliminates fear. Action fights stress. Action is the strategic sprint toward the solution.

Sprints can be just as beneficial in our personal lives as they are in our professional careers or fitness goals. A few years ago, Stef and I found out about a two-week therapy and counseling workshop for couples. We had a few friends attend before us, and they spoke very highly of the impact it made on their marriage and relationship. These two weeks were designed to reduce distractions from the outside world and hyper-focus on the couples. It allowed them to explore issues, discuss their problems, and improve their communication skills. The workshop is hosted on a farm, surrounded by beautiful scenery and a trained staff, participants are not allowed to have their phones with them, and everyone must completely remove themselves from their work during the retreat. While Stef and I haven't attended yet, we plan to in the future. It's an opportunity to go all in on our relationship and be proactive as we continue to build our family. This two-week therapy workshop focuses on specificity and intensity. It is a focused sprint with long-term potential for growth.

Our entire lives are a balance of proactive planning and intentional responding. There will be many situations that tempt us to react, but the goal is to respond. A response is a sign of maturity. It comes with practice and requires patience. Part of proactive planning is knowing when to incorporate sprints. These periods of time allow you to focus on less and do more. The specificity of these sprints facilitate refinement in all parts of our lives, including our fitness, our work, or even our personal relationships. While sprints aren't necessary, they can be a powerful tool to go all in on your mission with amplified intensity for short periods of time.

What We Want Versus What We Like

Being all in versus all consumed comes down to making deliberate choices. One thing to consider is that our decision-making is driven by the brain chemical dopamine, something I first mentioned in chapter 3. I was able to sit down with Daniel Z. Lieberman, one of the authors of the book *The Molecule of More,* and he shared how both choice and dopamine response control our ability to create progress in life. It's ultimately the act of discipline. While dopamine is a very powerful tool, powerful tools can be good and bad.

"A chainsaw can do great things. It can also do terrible things," Lieberman told me. "I think dopamine is largely responsible for all of the blessings we have today in terms of our technological society. These are all things that the development was driven by dopamine. But at the same time, dopamine doesn't have a brake. It never says enough. Dopamine always wants more and more and more. And so when we take things too far, the chemical that can save lives can also destroy lives."

The reality is what we want is not necessarily what we like. Our brains tell us we want certain things that we might not actually want for ourselves. Those wants may be influenced by social media, societal standards, or the desire to maintain a certain social status to keep up with our peers and community. The things we want are an imagination of the future. We assume those things will make us happier, but do they really? Usually not, because by the time we get them, they don't fulfill us like we thought they would. What we like is something we already have. It doesn't have to be

172 | GO ONE MORE

materialistic, although it may be. We know we like it because we have had time to experience it, play with it, use it, and incorporate it into our lifestyle. There is a real, true value associated with its use.

What we want is driven by dopamine, which is a neurotransmitter that is released that makes us desire future rewards, experiences, and achievements. It doesn't matter how much we have (food, money, material objects, successes, etc.), dopamine will always *want* more. Dopamine is not an inherently bad thing. It stimulates desire and motivation. It allows us to work, put forth effort, and chase our wildest aspirations, goals, and ambitions. But what happens when we finally get what we think we want? Are we fully satisfied, content, and fulfilled? Usually not. We want more. Why? Dopamine. Our wants don't always equate to what actually brings us joy and fulfillment in life. What brings us joy is driven by different brain chemicals: the Here and Now (H&N) neurotransmitters, which include serotonin, oxytocin, endorphins, and endocannabinoids. These brain chemicals allow us to appreciate the present moment.

Here's a story to illustrate this. In 2022, ten years after starting my business, I decided to treat myself with a ten-year business anniversary gift. I had worked hard, saved my money, and made financially smart decisions to the best of my ability, so I deserved and had earned a present. Right? At least this is what all the other entrepreneur gurus were telling me online. Then I saw it one day while driving down the road: a brand-new Chevy Corvette. So I went out and ordered it.

For months, all I could think about was this Corvette.

I'm going to drive it all the time, I thought. *It's so jacked up. It's going to change my life.* Six months after purchasing it, the Corvette arrived, fully loaded. It was beautiful. I took it for a drive and then parked it in the garage. The next day when I drove it to work, reality set in. I felt like an idiot driving it through town and stopping at intersections. It looked like the Batmobile. When I arrived at BPN, I parked in the back of the parking lot. I was actually embarrassed by it.

This is not me.

The Corvette was a lot, but it wasn't me. It made me feel all kinds of things, but none of them were cool, confident, or proud. Over the next couple weeks, I drove it less and less. I didn't drive it to work anymore because I was ashamed by it. I didn't even let anyone know I bought it. I put new wheels and tires on it, thinking that would make me more excited, but that didn't do a thing. Then I got it wrapped and put a body kit on it, thinking that would get me more inspired, but nothing changed. It didn't take long for me to realize that I actually didn't even like the Corvette.

So why did I buy it in the first place? Well, I wanted it. I really did. Yet when it finally came, I didn't like it—not one bit. As I think back to when I ordered the Corvette, I remember feeling overwhelmed with excitement. My brain was flooded with dopamine as I dropped off the deposit for the sports car and thought about how happy I was going to be as I drove it around town.

The reality is many of the things we think we want actually don't equate to the things we may like. The problem in so many of our lives is that we're chasing these wants. The key is finding balance between our wants and likes. As Lieberman wrote in *The Molecule of More*, "Too much dopamine can lead to productive misery, while too much H&N can lead to happy indolence."

In navigating the balance we have between dopamine and H&N—which is ultimately balancing all in versus all consumed—you have to be self-aware. It's easy to become all consumed by the things we want in the future. It leads to an obsession of never having enough and always wanting more and more and more. All consumed ignores H&N and is fully driven by dopamine, while all in recognizes both the H&N and dopamine. Being all in allows you to appreciate the present and identify things you like, but it's also driven by future possibilities and desires.

You have to be willing to have hard and honest conversations with yourself. The word "balance" takes a lot of shame. It's something many people want, but very few believe is achievable. I think many of us need to redefine our meaning of balance, myself included. Balance isn't an on-off switch where we get to teeter between work and pleasure. It's more so like a dimmer switch that is driven by seasons and sprints, between ambition and contentment. Dopamine drives our ambition. It wants more. More achievement. More success. More wins. H&N drives our contentment. Enjoying the silence of an evening walk. Sitting at dinner with friends and family. Drinking coffee on the front porch with your spouse. I aim to be all in on creating a balanced life rather than all consumed by the drive for more dopamine.

I'm a pretty impulsive person. I've become less impulsive over the years, but it still gets me in trouble from time to time. Impulsive decisions and actions are usually driven by dopamine. And I, just like many of you, am a dopamine junkie. I love it. But as I've become more aware of its downfalls, I've also learned how to control the dopamine desire of more. Now, when I feel the dopamine being released into my brain and I begin to want something, I sit on it. I wait. I consider the benefits and consequences. I think about how it will make me feel initially and then down the road. I try to distinguish between my desire for and satisfaction with this want. If it is something that, after much thought, time, and consideration, I still want, then I will pursue it. But only after I'm fairly certain it will produce just as much like as want. This fuels the clarity required to fully implement Go One More.

Flip the Switch

It is never too late to flip the switch and shift from being all consumed to being all in. This is something I have had to do, especially since becoming a father.

I learned a hard lesson about all in versus all consumed the last time I did a bodybuilding prep. Unlike the marathon preps I had done before that, the prep for my bodybuilding competition in 2023 was all-consuming. I underestimated how hard the training and diet would be because the last time I trained for a competition, in 2012, I didn't have all the extra responsibilities I now had. It is brutal when you restrict calories to a certain point, your energy is depleted, your hormones are impeded, and your metabolic health is a wreck. You're thinking about the next meal and what you can eat while you're getting leaner and tighter to step on stage. It is the very definition of all-consuming; you think about it from the moment you wake up to the time you go to sleep. It distracts you from every other aspect of your life. And as the competition date gets closer and closer, the all-consuming mentality becomes worse and worse. Every calorie is accounted for, the scale and body fat percentage take over your mind, and body dysmorphia controls you.

I respect the sport and the people who do bodybuilding, but I decided that the competition in 2023 would be my last. I was all consumed, and to be honest, it is a horrible lifestyle for someone who previously struggled with a severe eating disorder. My mind was constantly thinking about calories, macronutrients, body weight, fat loss, and training. I was committed to seeing the goal through, but the process was destroying my life and my relationships with people who meant the most to me. That didn't fit the life I want, and it didn't align with the priorities I was setting out to live and achieve.

Sometimes, there is a firm line between all in and all consumed, a line that is not blurry or muddy at all. A line that you know you cross when you are all consumed. The peak of my eating disorder was all-consuming. I needed control over everything in order to feel safe and secure. Fitness goals and journeys can be all-consuming. It's the moment that a healthy habit becomes an unhealthy one. There was a moment during my bodybuilding prep in 2023 when I knew I crossed the line.

We were out to dinner with friends one night in

Georgetown, Texas. It was a popular Tex-Mex restaurant that we loved. I really didn't want to go out for dinner because it forced me to eat foods that I didn't prepare and couldn't accurately track calorically. When the waiter came around to take our orders, I asked how the chicken fajitas were prepared. He explained to me that they were pre-marinated in an oil-based dressing and then cooked on a grill top with oil. I really didn't want to be difficult, but I politely asked if they could rinse the chicken under water prior to cooking it on the grill. Trust me, I know how ridiculous this sounds. To my surprise, he was more than happy to make that happen for me, and I appreciated that. When our food arrived, which I was already stressed about, my chicken looked like it was dripping in oil. I said nothing and began wiping my chicken down with wet napkins and drying them on a separate plate. Again, to reinforce, bodybuilding prep will do crazy things to your mind. Inside I was fuming. My mind was spiraling. I thought:

This is going to throw my entire prep off track.

I'm going to gain body fat from this meal.

I should've just brought my own food to the restaurant.

Meanwhile, as I'm trying to recover the health integrity of this poor chicken breast, I looked over to my daughter, who was about six months old at the time, and saw her watching me. I felt ashamed and embarrassed. *Is this the message I'm teaching my child? Am I showing her that this is okay? Will she inherit disordered eating from me?* I knew in that moment that I had crossed the line. I was all consumed.

When I flipped from being all consumed to all in, I was able to focus on my responsibilities as opposed to just routines. It forced me to be intentional with my decisions, my time, and my obligations. Flipping the switch allowed me to focus on my meaningful mission in life, so flip the switch now.

You might be asking yourself, *Where is this switch? What do I need to do to go from being all consumed to all in? What do I need to change?*

When you are all in, you've discovered clarity. Your thoughts, intentions, and motivations are clear. The previous chapters have explained exactly what you need to change in order to be all in. It starts with having awareness of where you are, where you want to be, and how you are going to get there. It starts with proving yourself right. When you are working toward a goal to prove to yourself that you can do it, you will focus on being all in. However, when you are concerned with the opinions, criticism, and doubt from other people, you will be all consumed with proving them wrong.

Being all in is settling into the driver's seat of life and enduring the process. It's not being consumed by the outcomes or focused on being occasionally great, but it is showing up consistently and putting in the work to get better. Those who are all in can appreciate delayed gratification. They will go further for the love of the journey and not the destination.

As I was working through this section of the book, I asked my wife what she has seen me do when I've flipped the switch. By asking that question, I realized the importance of having someone in your life who will tell you when you are all consumed by something. That's what Stef does for me, even when I see it, too. She's open and honest with me, and after it's addressed, we talk about it. To flip the switch, I begin with identifying what matters to me. Just as I discussed in chapter 5, if something matters to you, you will make time. Then I align what matters to me with my schedule. They should reflect one another. From there, I ensure my responsibilities are prioritized over my routines.

That's how you flip the switch. You can flip that switch right now.

Don't Clear Your Head, Find Clarity

How do you find the balance between all in and all consumed? How do you know when to sprint and when to flip the switch? How can you balance the ambition that is driven by dopamine while also being content in the here and now?

It comes down to clarity. This book is ultimately about gaining and achieving clarity through these lessons and perspectives in order to implement Go One More. To do that, you need understand what clarity really is and how to achieve it.

My running coach Jeff Cunningham said that a lot of people say they're going to run to "clear their head," but he believes that's not really what they want. People don't run or meditate or sit in a sauna to clear their head. They do these things to gain clarity. There's a difference between clearing your head and gaining clarity. When you clear your head, your mind is empty. This can be good or bad, but I don't think it's super beneficial. On the other hand, when you try to achieve and gain clarity, your thoughts and mind are organized thoughts. Without that mental clarity, our minds are busy and noisy, and we can be self-destructive as a result.

I've had many self-destructive days and times of my life. Even though I'm aware of these things, it still happens to me, and it's likely still going to happen to everyone. But the solution is to be aware. So we need to define the difference between clearing your mind and clarity and emphasize why clarity is so important. It is pure organization. This clarity is the reason I run. When I run, and I'm achieving and gaining clarity, I have organized thoughts that allow me to plan and strategize more intentionally.

All the concepts in this book—especially being all in instead of all consumed—are about mitigating the risk of self-destruction. So many people end up being self-destructive at some point in their lives, and it's often why they don't achieve their goals. It's why they don't accomplish the things they set out to. I don't think failure is typically the result of external factors. It's not a catastrophic tornado or death in the family or a traumatic experience. The reason most people don't achieve the things they want to and set out to achieve is self-destruction. For me, what self-destruction looks like is a lack of organized thoughts. Not having clarity.

In his book *Deep Work: Rules for Focused Success in a Distracted World*, Cal Newport explores the idea of clarity. So often, we want our lives to be busier. We want to be doing more. We are seduced by hustle culture that tells us to constantly search for something so we can gain an edge or get to the next level, even though it's not necessarily productive. Newport encourages readers to find opportunities in areas of solitude, presence, and quietness to eliminate distractions, stop being busy, and just be present. Because when you are present, you're going to make up so much ground. Your mind will be clear, and you will be able to focus on your meaningful mission. "Clarity about what matters provides clarity about what does not," Newport wrote.

When I am running, I am able to unlock parts of my brain and find clarity that is unavailable to me when I'm sitting at my desk for three hours. For some people, that is productive, but not for me. I will find ways to distract myself. I will think of everything other than deep work. I need to be actively moving or doing something to think very deeply.

Running is my solution to find clarity. It might be for you as well, but if it's not, I encourage you to search for a routine time and place that promotes solitude. The clarity you will experience in those moments of solitude will allow you to audit your life and ensure you are all in rather than all consumed. Find time in your day to carve out these moments, even if it's for a few short minutes. These moments matter.

Chapter Seven

DOUBT IS ONLY DANGEROUS WHEN YOU START DOUBTING YOURSELF

"Don't act so surprised. Unbelievable happens all the time. Sometimes it's divine, and sometimes it's a loogie in our face. Don't deny it. Depend on it, expect it. Believe it."
—Matthew McConaughey, *Greenlights*

Y ou are the only person who needs to believe.

It took me a long time to learn this, and I had to learn it the hard way. When you announce that there is something bold and difficult you want to achieve, the world and people around you will let you know how likely you are to fail. Sometimes this is your best friend, a stranger, a family member, or someone observing your life from social media. Since day one of starting my business, I was doubted. When I announced certain physical feats I wanted to accomplish, I was doubted. That doubt had no impact on my ability to achieve success; however, it could have if I had started doubting myself. I don't share this to position myself as a victim of doubters and critics. We all have people in our lives, whether they make it publicly known or not, that are rooting against us. And that's perfectly fine as long as we don't allow them to influence our ability to take massive action.

The moment I realized the power of this way of thinking, my life changed. Many great and successful people have changed the trajectory of the world through a strong belief in themselves, even when no one else believed. Imagine the number of people who could have reached their full potential but never did because they bought into the doubt of others. One comment, one opinion, one opposing perspective has the power to change the trajectory of your life if you allow it. Draw a line in the sand right now. Don't let that happen.

Do you find it challenging to show up as your authentic self? Do self-doubt and personal insecurity hold you back from living out an authentic, genuine, and fulfilling life? I have been there. I have said and done things that didn't represent me. I have made decisions even when my intuition was begging me not to. I have been insecure about my eating disorder in the past. I have hesitated because of my lack of business knowledge and experience in the early days of BPN. I have been distracted by the criticism I received when sharing my life with the world. Once I realized that those insecurities provided me no benefit, no advantage, and no fulfillment, I started becoming more vulnerable and honest with myself.

A few years ago, I had Matt Beaudreau on my podcast. He was once a professor at Stanford University until he realized that the education system was broken, and he made it his life's mission to fix it. I had a lightbulb moment with Matt that has stuck with me ever since. I asked him, from his perspective, what mistake most parents make while raising children and young adults. He responded, "They outsource everything." Bingo. That's it. That was once my problem and the thought process that holds so many people back from achieving greatness. Not just parents. Everyone. We outsource our thoughts, ideas, opinions, and perspectives to other people so we can then adopt an inauthentic self that is a reflection of experts and gurus of who knows what.

I realized that doubt is only dangerous when you start doubting yourself. When we allow doubt and insecurity to consume us, we quickly begin to lose hope. But if we are confident in our ability to overcome any obstacles that stand in our way, we won't quit until the battle is won. We don't have to outsource everything. Delegate parts? Yes. But outsource? No.

This chapter explores the doubts and fears we all have. Fear and anxiety are normal emotions tied to the pursuit of great things, but at your core, you must always believe in your abilities. End your pursuit of perfection and find a victory in finishing something. Stop comparing yourself to others. Instead, say that nothing is ever unbelievable. Block out any outside noise and control what is yours to control. Belief in one's self is the most powerful tool we can harness because belief is resilient, adaptable, and relentless during denial.

Your Gut Is Calibrated

I've made some of my worst decisions, lost significant amounts of money, and thrown my life off course multiple times by neglecting my gut. Our gut, also known as our intuition, is calibrated from years of experience, exposure, and repetition. With more experience, age, and wisdom, our gut decisions become stronger and better and lead us to a greater likelihood of success. It's like artificial intelligence; our gut gets smarter on its own after years and years of calibration.

In 2023, I made a decision that neglected my gut's intuition and turned my life upside down for the next fifteen months. I stepped down from the CEO role of BPN and moved into a chief creative officer role, primarily focused on brand awareness. Why? I doubted my ability to take the business to the next level while also being the husband and father I wanted to be. I didn't think I had the skills, experience, or capacity to lead the business to do it all. I wasn't confident in my ability to be that leader. Some of these insecurities were internally created, but others were influenced by respected people in my life. I was told that it was "time to hire a professional operator" and that "I did a great job getting the business to this point, but it now required some-one with greater industry experience to scale it." It seemed like a lot of people doubted me as the CEO, leader, and op-erator of the business. It also felt like my abilities to be the family man I wanted and needed to be were being doubted as well. And when enough people start doubting you, it's easy to start doubting yourself. That was one of the greatest mistakes I made, and it cost me.

Shortly after I stepped down from the CEO role, we launched a formal process with an investment bank (the private equity deal I discussed in chapter 4). The goal was to bring on a private equity partner that would invest a sig-nificant amount of money and own a minority share in the business. A large portion of that investment was to be dis-tributed to shareholders, and I was the largest shareholder. A smaller portion of that investment was to be distributed to BPN's balance sheet and bank account. The waterfall of those funds would have meant that I would exchange a portion of my equity in BPN for life-changing money. But the doubt that I had in myself earlier that year caught up to me in a meaningful way.

We worked hard to get the private equity deal across the finish line for about a year, and after all was said and done, days before the funds were going to be sent, the deal fell apart. I received the call from the managing director of the investment bank we had been working with at 10 PM on a Wednesday night. And just like that, the process we had been working toward and were 99.9 percent confident was going to get done was over.

So, where did I go wrong? Just like Matt Beaudreau said,

I outsourced the wrong things. I stepped out of the driver's seat and let other people control the outcomes of my life and business. While many people doubted my ability, I knew deep down in my core that I was the right person to take my business to the next level. But as that doubt slowly transitioned from other people to myself, the dangers of disbelief sank in. I ignored my intuition and stopped trusting my gut, which had been calibrated to make the right choice over the previous decade.

In Bedros Keuilian's book *Man Up*, he talks about how detrimental self-doubt can be. "The negative belief system is crippling. Your beliefs dictate your habits. Habits dictate actions. Actions dictate outcomes. Belief is everything."

Just as Keuilian shares, everything we achieve or fail to achieve starts with belief. It is the foundation of what we pursue or choose to let die. If you continue to doubt your ability to accomplish the things you want to do, you will never get there. You will probably never even get started. Confidence and belief in one's self grows with preparation and practice, but sometimes you just have to wake up, look in the mirror, and tell yourself you are going to do the damn thing. Then go do it. I'm not talking about positive self-talk or affirmations. I'm talking about owning the outcome. Own your life. Don't let someone else own it for you.

When I started my business, some people made fun of me. I said I was going to do something, and then I went and did it. That challenged a lot of other people's courage to do the same. But if I would have let that belief control my narrative, my thought process, and my security, there is no way I would be where I am today. Thankfully I didn't buy into that belief early on. Everyone can doubt you and say whatever they want, but until you actually start believing what they're saying, you remain in the driver's seat. Or as Keuilian says, you're flying the fighter jet. "You could very easily, if you start believing what the doubters say, turn that fighter jet into a crop duster that is not worthy of going to battle and winning the spoils."

So many might see an entrepreneur like Bedros Keuilian or myself and think, *There's no way I can do what you've done. I'm not a high performer.* But there is no secret formula or special ability. A thousand people might tell you you're going to fail, but none of that will impact you unless you let those seeds take root in your mind. When you do that, it's over before it can even begin.

So what are some examples of those seeds of doubt? Comparison and perfectionism are two common ones.

The Difference between Unhealthy Comparison and Healthy Inspiration

More than ever before, we compare ourselves to others, judging their skills and achievements against our own. With the advancements in technology, social media, and our increasingly interconnected lives, I can't imagine it getting much better unless we make intentional choices to resist the constant temptation of comparison.

If there was one thing you could eliminate today that would greatly benefit your life, happiness, fulfillment, and purpose, it would be unhealthy comparison. It's toxic. Some may argue that it's competitive, and it can be, but I would counter that, generally, it's not healthy competition. We compare our success, financial status, social media follower count, physical bodies, material possessions, and athletic abilities to other people, most of whom we don't know and will never meet. I'm not saying I've never been guilty of this, but I'm now self-aware enough to know when I'm comparing myself in an unhealthy way and when I'm not. I know when it's causing good, healthy competitive behavior and when it's destructive in all forms. Even when we know it's destructive, however, we often still allow it to swirl around our minds a few times before making a reactive decision driven by dopamine.

One of my favorite sayings is "You can't compare your chapter one to someone else's chapter ten." It's so true, yet we all fall victim to it no matter how many times we hear the words. The earlier chapters of each journey we embark on are some of the best ones in the book. They are filled with ignorance, naiveté, and a "burn the boats" mentality to jump all the way in and get started. Those are the intimidating days, the unknown months, and the most challenging yet rewarding years. Be proud of those times. Embrace the humbling days. Be confident in what you know, but be more honest with what you don't. Ask for help and don't apologize for where you are and what you are doing. Don't doubt or downplay your goals, operation, or traction. Stand tall and upright as you proudly talk about where you're heading. The North Star. That's your chapter ten, twenty, thirty, forty, fifty, and so on.

I've made the most progress in my personal and professional life when I've kept my head down and focused on building my business, my fitness, my body, and my team and family. This head down time is about focus. It eliminates the distraction of comparison and ultimately helps you maintain your trajectory toward your North Star.

———————

When I started seriously running and training for races, I was embarrassed by my lack of endurance. I would find myself on the Lady Bird Lake loop in downtown Austin, running at paces I could barely hold just to keep up with the runners around me. People I followed on social media would post photos of their races, splits, training paces, heart rates, and all of the other data points that reinforced my fear of being "slow." I vividly remember finishing some of my earlier runs feeling great, looking strong, and getting faster just to be crushed after seeing the results someone else posted on social media. Same distances, faster paces, lower heart rate, easier effort.

I suck.

I'm just not made to be a runner.

Bigger-boned. Larger frame. I'll never be fast.

And for a split second in time, I started to believe it. I began to doubt myself. That doubt lived for a minute before I crushed its ability to thrive. Sometimes I think about what I would be doing and where I would be if I had allowed that doubt to prevent me from pursuing my full potential.

But it's just running, right?

At face value, yes. But running has changed my life. It created a space for me to think deeply. It has been the silence and solitude I needed to show up intentionally for my work, my family, and myself. This passion, which my wife may consider an obsession, has changed the course of my business, reach, and story. Running is my clarity. It facilitates the outcome of Go One More.

After realizing the negative impact that comparing my running performance had been creating, I chose a different strategy. I stopped comparing my running journey to anyone else's. I would love to tell you I did this because I was proactive enough to realize I had crossed the line from inspiration to comparison, but that's not the case. To be honest, comparison is exhausting. It's debilitating. I made the conscious effort and decision to channel my energy toward a strategy that left me more fulfilled rather than empty, more excited rather than resentful. Choosing inspiration over comparison is a personal responsibility. You get to decide what you consume and what you do with it. If you are constantly comparing yourself to others—your chapter one to someone else's chapter ten, or even your "easy run" to a professional athlete's data points—it's because you have put yourself in that position. Ending the comparison saga requires you to eliminate the source and loosen the hold it has on your wrist.

Now, as much as I'm an advocate of staying focused and minimizing comparison, I have to acknowledge that sometimes it can be helpful to look to the success of others as inspiration. Austin Kleon illustrates this idea in his book *Steal Like an Artist*, a guide to creativity that encourages readers to pull inspiration from the people, brands, and teams that are doing it the best. It's an amazing book and a short, easy read. Kleon says that nothing is original, so embrace influence, school yourself through the work of others, and mix and reimagine to discover your own path. From the way I understand Austin's work, he isn't suggesting that we compare what we are doing, creating, or building to the work of others, but we should watch, listen, and learn from the work of others to influence our ability to create our best work possible.

"You're only going to be as good as the stuff you surround yourself with," Kleon wrote. "My mom used to say to me, 'Garbage in, garbage out.' It used to drive me nuts. But now I know what she meant. Your job is to collect ideas. The more good ideas you collect, the more you can choose from to be influenced by."

Now I'm not suggesting you lock yourself in your room and work toward your goal in confined solitude. You would go crazy. And I'm not telling you to create boundaries that shield you from others' work in the outside world. That inspiration is necessary. But my goal with this message is to highlight the difference between unhealthy comparison and healthy inspiration. Unhealthy comparison makes you feel bad about yourself; it drives self-doubt and causes you to become resentful, bitter, and angry. On the flip side, healthy inspiration sparks creativity; it ignites optimism and enthusiasm. It is the passion and motivation required to work toward achieving the goal.

We are never the best versions of ourselves when we are comparing our success to others. I know because I've been there more times than I'd like to admit. I've created narratives in my head about how horrible a person is all because they were ahead of me. Their business was larger, their performance was stronger, their races were faster, or their bodies were leaner. I turned them into enemies just because, by comparing myself to them, I felt inferior. It never felt good, and eventually I realized that by maintaining that attitude, I couldn't be the leader, father, or husband I wanted to be. It wasn't a legacy I would be proud of, and it didn't align with Go One More.

While inspiration can take you further than you thought possible, remember that comparison is usually unhealthy. It is the root of self-doubt. Realize that your journey is unique. Your process is unfolding at a necessary rate, one that allows you to gain important experience, acquire knowledge, and progress into a greater version of yourself.

Nothing Is Unbelievable

At the end of the early 2000s, Matthew McConaughey was one of the biggest and most bankable actors in Hollywood. He was the go-to guy for romantic comedies such as *How to Lose a Guy in 10 Days* and *The Wedding Planner*. He enjoyed making them, but after being in the film industry for fifteen years, McConaughey decided to make a change. The rom-coms felt too easy and safe for him. He wanted to do more challenging roles in dramas. So he called his agent and took the biggest risk he had ever taken in his career. The industry, however, had other ideas.

In an interview I had with him about his book *Greenlights*, McConaughey shared, "Industry says, 'No, thank you. Not you, McConaughey. We don't care how much of a pay cut you would take. We're not hiring you for those.'" He ultimately decided to cut out the romantic comedies and adventure comedies altogether, knowing it was a huge risk since that was his lane, a lane that not only fed him but also fed Hollywood. He knew he was going to be out of work for a while, but he wasn't sure how long it would be.

"I was taking a one-way ticket into the limbo of not knowing, and I didn't know how long it would go on," McConaughey told me. "After a year, I thought, *Man, I may have written my one-way ticket out of Hollywood. Hollywood may have just given me that middle finger.*"

But for months, he held the course. He would call his agent and ask if there was anything, but he soon realized that nobody was mentioning his name. *They forgot about me,* McConaughey thought. *I'm done.* His wife was there to keep him stable over the long days of feeling insignificant, and he severely doubted what future opportunities would come in Hollywood, but he never doubted himself.

"I was like, 'Hang on, stick to this, stick to this. I'll endure this. Pay the penance, whatever it is.' Nineteen months go by. I'm not even thinking about Hollywood anymore. I'm ready to go start coaching a middle school football team and maybe work my way up to a high school coach or something. I'm thinking I'm going to do something else with my life. Then the phone rings."

Suddenly, the industry had a novel idea to have him star in a dramatic role. McConaughey had been gone long enough for people to find some anonymity. The world hadn't seen him in a romantic comedy for years. What came next was a series of roles in films that led to what the industry called

"McConaissance" and him eventually winning an Academy Award for Best Actor in a Leading Role in the film *Dallas Buyers Club*.

"Look, I had moments and moments of doubt," McConaughey said. "But underneath it all, I had a true belief that, hey, I've got the goods to do the work that I wanted."

During our conversation, I asked McConaughey about a quote I heard him say about how "unbelievable" was the most foolish word in the dictionary.

"Unbelievable—it doesn't give justice to the awesomeness of a situation or the degradation. It's a default word that nips off how high the ceiling can be and nips off how low the basement."

People use the word "unbelievable" all the time to describe both triumphs and tragedies in our world. How could something like a musical performance be "unbelievable" even though we just witnessed it and it was awesome?

"I'm a proponent of extending the bandwidth, of giving credit to things that are absolutely awe-inspiring and incredible in life, and extending the bandwidth down low to the things that are ugly in life but true in life, whether they're from Mother Nature or whether they're from mankind," McConaughey said. "And so many of the things that humans do that are awesome or absolutely ugly and evil, we should give those credit and look them in the eye, not slap them as being unbelievable. It's a silly habit for us to throw 'unbelievable' around so much because it just doesn't give enough credit to where credit needs to be given."

It's funny how one interaction, one conversation, can change the way you think about one thing for the rest of your entire life. That conversation forever changed how I think about the word "unbelievable." I sometimes catch myself about to finish a sentence with the word and I stop and replace it with something else. When you position something, someone, an event, or a moment in history as unbelievable, you are discrediting its realness and power to do great or destructive things. What is truly unbelievable? I don't think any of us really know. God knows, but with each year, the human race pushes the boundaries of what was once impossible. As soon as we tag something as unbelievable, we are not only doubting its ability to be done, but our ability to be the one who does it. That doubt is dangerous on its own, and as long as it exists, everything it occupies will be unbelievable.

Fail Forward

I truly believe we should all set "hard" physical goals every single year. I put hard in quotations because that word is relative. What is hard for you might not be hard for me and vice versa. Regardless, we need to do hard things because, in its absence, we atrophy, become weak, and die. That doesn't only apply to our bodies, but also our minds and spirits. Hard objectives keep us sharp and honest with ourselves. It has to be hard enough so we are required to fight. It shouldn't come easy or as a guarantee. It should be hard enough to break you but also build you into someone you wouldn't have been without the experience. Former US President Teddy Roosevelt described the results we receive from these opportunities in his speech at the Sorbonne:

The credit belongs to the man who is actually in the arena, whose face is marred by dust and sweat and blood, who strives valiantly, who errs and comes up short again and again, because there is no effort without error or short-coming, but who knows the great enthusiasms, the great devotions, who spends himself for a worthy cause; who, at the best, knows in the end, the triumph of high achievement, and who at the worst, if he fails, at least he fails while daring greatly, so that his place shall never be with those cold and timid souls who knew neither victory nor defeat.

So, why should we choose hard things?

First off, it's humbling, and those encounters build a greater layer of self-awareness that reinforces self-account-ability. Every time I go after an ambitious, hard physical goal, I'm always reminded how much better I can be by how fast the process of improvement breaks me. Challenging work-outs, long training days, and preps that last a few months will show you just how committed you are to the outcome. And when it's time to be tested, the "arena" will either pro-vide you a fighting chance or chew you up and spit you out if you aren't prepared for the challenge. Success isn't guaran-teed, and failure may be more likely than we want to believe, but if we're going to fail, we must fail forward. We need to identify our weaknesses, our struggles, and our limitations because, in the absence of self-awareness, we start to believe perfection is possible in an imperfect world.

Second, sometimes we need to feel inferior. In Ichiro Kishimi's book *The Courage to be Disliked*, he talks about the difference between feelings of being inferior and an inferiority complex. They are much different. "A healthy feeling of being inferior is not something that comes from comparing oneself to others; it comes from one's comparison with one's ideal self," Kishimi wrote.

When we have healthy feelings of being inferior, it keeps us pushing forward. It generates ambition, drive, and the desire to reach our greatest potential in life. Feelings of being inferior are why we, as human beings, continue to evolve throughout time. That feeling generates questions of:

What else am I capable of?

How can I do this better?

How can I be the best?

What do I need to do to improve?

Having an inferiority complex, however, is not so beneficial for you or the people around you. An inferiority complex is an intense personal feeling of inadequacy and often leads one to compare their physical attributes, mental limitations, or differences in social status to that of others. Feelings of being inferior push us toward greatness, while an inferiority complex buries us in self-doubt and destruction.

The third reason we should set a hard goal every year is because it builds confidence. In my opinion, one of society's greatest faults is that many people lack self-confidence, have low self-esteem, and honestly strongly dislike who they are. Confidence doesn't happen on its own or get better with age. It requires intentional work to build and maintain. Setting goals, establishing a plan, working toward those goals, and accomplishing them builds confidence. With more repetition comes more confidence, but also more losses along the way. You will fail. We all fail. Failure is good as long as we learn from it. The more wins you stack in life, the larger your self-confidence builds.

I first heard about the concept of the Misogi from entrepreneur, author, and musician Jesse Itzler. The Misogi is an ancient Japanese practice that embraces physical and mental challenges to help one gain a deeper understanding of themself by pushing beyond their limits and building confidence, self-awareness, and strength. The Misogi, however, should truly be a challenge. It should be something hard enough that doesn't guarantee success. If you're crossing the finish line every time, you need to set greater goals. Every year, Jesse puts one year-defining event on his calendar. This could be publishing a book, running a one-hundred-mile race, launching a podcast, or becoming a private pilot. Everyone needs a Misogi, he says. I agree, and I think a hard physical goal is one of the best ways to approach it. So choose your hard thing. Choose wisely. And get to work.

I personally couldn't imagine a life where I'm not pushing myself hard physically in some capacity every single year. When we choose hard things, it leads us toward a better life. Not an easier life, but a life full of more opportunities. More fulfillment. More experiences. More growth. These hardships ultimately expose our weaknesses, so because of this, we are given a roadmap for where we can best spend our time to get better. But aren't all of these hard things stressful on the body? Absolutely; that's the point. Stress is a requirement for growth. Stress facilitates an adaptation for growth and development. The mind and body build in a similar way as a single muscle fiber does. When we train, the stimulus we endure creates micro-tears, damage, and necessary destruction to our muscle fibers. What happens next is adaptation. Over the following days, our bodies work to heal and repair the damaged muscle fibers, and through that process, they become increasingly bigger, stronger, more durable, and more adaptable than before. That stress is a requirement for improvement. Don't run away from it. Don't avoid it. Run toward it. Embrace it.

Without hard challenges, placing ourselves in the "arena," and failing, we will continue to question our true capabilities. We will doubt what can be done because we aren't willing to find out due to fear of failure. The only way to eliminate the fear of failure is by action. Do more, fail more, but fail forward. As long as we hold back because we are afraid to miss the goal and be marked as a failure, our potential will be capped and self-doubt will control our lives.

Choose Your Superpowers

What comes to mind when you think of a superhero? Many times, we think of someone who can fly, turn back time, or shoot webs out of his wrists. We think of flashy physical traits and abilities that serve a very specific purpose. For me, when I picture a superhero, I think of someone who is strong, confident, brave, courageous, selfless, and tough. Real traits that exist in mortal beings. The great part about life is that you are in control of choosing your superpowers. And there are five superpowers that I think can change the trajectory of somebody's life: self-accountability, consistency, courage, curiosity, and toughness. These superpowers are a determining factor for character, ability, willpower, and discipline, and they are the superpowers that I am constantly trying to capture and refine.

Occasionally, when I'm overwhelmed, overworked, and stressed, I have this thought process where I pull out of the body I'm in and view myself from a third-person perspective. In that moment, I realize, *Nick, you are in control. You are in control of implementing and utilizing the superpowers that you have created and refined for years and years and years. So put them to work. Deploy your superpowers.*

Life moves fast and things change. As the ancient Greek philosopher Epictetus said, "It's not what happens to you, but how you react to it that matters." How you react is determined by the tools you have that can be applied to the problem you're trying to solve. We can add an unmeasurable number of tools to our kit, but there only will be a few that you use regularly. Think of a general contractor's tool collection. There is something for everything. But there are a few tools that the contractor uses daily, like a hammer, screwdriver, or tape measure. Those tools are the superpowers for that tradesperson's job. Similarly, you get to choose the superpowers you collect, refine, and deploy. Don't let anyone tell you otherwise. There are two superpowers I want to hone in on here because they work hand-in-hand: courage and curiosity.

Why are people unhappy? Why do so many in our society find themselves feeling unfulfilled? Why are we so lonely? It's because of a lack of courage. Maybe you think courage has nothing to do with being unhappy and unfulfilled, but here is the reason it does: a lack of courage holds us back from accomplishing all of our dreams and aspirations. Courage is action; it's taking that first step. You can have all the confidence in the world, but confidence is a belief. Courage, on the other hand, is the action taken on that belief. The result of courage is momentum, and it allows the questions of your curiosity to be answered.

What is the reason people don't lose weight even if they desperately want to? It's the lack of courage. Same with the reason people are unhappy and unfulfilled. Courage propels the action needed to make a change. I could have wished all day that I was going to run a sub–2:40 marathon, but unless I had the courage to take the steps to make that happen, nothing would have changed. I can say I want my business to be worth $1 billion, but if I don't have the courage to put a plan in place, hire the right people, and have the work ethic required to get there, it's just a dream. It's just a wish. Real courage is a superpower that you can harness for a lot of great things.

Retired Navy SEAL Chadd Wright and I discussed courage on my podcast, and he said that most people tend to lose courage for what has to be done through the pursuit of the process, especially after struggling and failing.

"Every single one of us human beings—you're going to have to walk through these big piles of crap," Wright told me. "And there's probably going to be a bunch of them, right? So what happens in life when you do something stupid and you create this pile of crap and you have no other way to go but through it? You're walking through this crap, and it's getting deep, and it's getting hard, and it's painful, and it starts to get right up to your neck. A lot of people stop right there in the middle of that pile of crap and they never make it out the other side."

Some of those who do make it through that crap, Wright explained, end up carrying that shame for the rest of their lives. They hide in the corner and never try anything again. They never try to put themselves in environments where they feel uncomfortable. Regret and shame can stop a lot of people.

"There's been so many times in my life I've made so many mistakes," Wright said. "I've gotten covered in so much crap. And everybody looked at me and said, 'You are a freakin' turd.' And I said, 'Yeah, I am a turd. But guess what? I'm going to keep going, man.'"

This is what courage looks like. Continuing to move on and forgetting what you did ten years ago or ten months ago or even yesterday that might keep you stuck in place. Courage comes down to being able to answer a question, one that seems so basic but is also so complex that a lot of people have a hard time putting it into practice.

What do you want? What *don't* you want? What do you want your life to look like? Do you want to be happy? If you want to be happy, do you have the courage to make a change? If you're unhappy, something has to change. The change might come from changing the way you think, or it might come in the way you do something, but either way, it requires courage. So ask yourself what you want. It might seem like a really easy question to answer, but if you actually sit down and audit your life, what will you write down? What do you want your life to feel like? To look like? What do you want the experience to be like? Write that down and then have the courage to take the steps to make it happen.

The other superpower to embrace is curiosity. Now, curiosity without courage is useless. Just because you are curious about something doesn't mean anything. Nothing will change unless you act upon that curiosity, and that action is the courage to take that first step. So why don't we act on our curiosities? It comes back to those doubts we have. It's our fears that prevent us from acting on them.

Curiosity is the spark that makes us do the things we do. I would have never started my business if I wasn't curious. I would have never started running marathons if I wasn't curious. I would have never wanted to join the military, go through Ranger School, and be an infantry platoon leader if I wasn't curious. I would have never scaled my business to the size it is today if I wasn't curious. I would have never run a sub–2:39 marathon if I wasn't curious.

Sometimes we don't act on our curiosities because of our self-doubt and lack of courage. Other times, these doubts and fears come from other people. Have you ever had a curiosity and wanted to act on it, but then started to talk to someone or a group of people who instantly became pessimistic? People who highlighted what could go wrong, what things to be cautious about, and everything you should be afraid of? These doubts and fears they have start to jump from them onto you like bedbugs, and as soon as they get to you, they spread. You lose the courage to act and you shelve your curiosity.

We have to have the courage to be curious. We can't let ourselves or others spread the bedbugs of fear and doubt inside us. Don't let the fears of others influence your courage to act on your curiosity. Be fearless. Be truly fearless. And in doing so, be open-minded. This is something I've worked on the past couple years of my life that has opened my mind and perspective so much. It increases your perspective capacity. There are so many things happening in the world today, and we can't simply stay in our echo chamber where everyone believes exactly what you believe, thinks the exact same way you think, and likes exactly what you want and like. We need to be curious about other perspectives, values, and sides. When you remove the echo chamber and allow yourself to consume information from different people of varying backgrounds, perspectives, beliefs, and walks of life with an open mind, you add to your ability to be more curious. It can be a superpower you can harness and use. Being closed-minded will truly shut you off from growth potential. Not just professionally, but personally as well.

Courage and curiosity are truly two of the greatest superpowers you can harness. Without curiosity, we would never dream of building our businesses, chasing down our fitness goals, traveling the world, or wanting more in life. That curiosity releases dopamine that produces the desire, but we have to act on that desire with courage. Courage is the pursuit and exploration of the curiosity. You can't have one without the other.

Curiosity on its own may spark some doubt. It's normal, but it can also be dangerous. Be courageous enough to take action and believe in yourself to do whatever it is you want to do. Be courageous enough to ignore the doubt from others, and be confident in your ability because belief always comes before ability.

They Will Call You Crazy

Before Michael Hardy, known professionally as HARDY, was a famous singer/performer, he was a successful songwriter, and his career in country music appeared to be extremely promising. I was personally a fan of HARDY's music before his album release in 2023, but in all honesty, most of his music felt like just another bunch of hit radio songs. That's not to say there is anything wrong with that. His songs were catchy, easy listening, and had a good tune. I enjoyed them. But when he released *The Mockingbird & the Crow* in 2023, everything changed. Not just for me as a fan, but also for his career and position in the music industry. He is living proof that doubt is only dangerous when you start doubting yourself.

At the 15th Annual Academy of Country Music (ACM) Awards, HARDY received the ACM Songwriter of the Year award. During his acceptance speech, he told the story about how, at a show he played seven years earlier, he received a napkin in a tip jar with the word "quit" on it. Someone in the crowd that night was so displeased with his performance that they encouraged him to give up. To quit. To stop pursuing greatness because they doubted him so much. If HARDY would have believed this doubt as much as that person who left the napkin did, he would have never reached the level of success he has today. He would have missed out on opportunities, wins, setbacks, experiences, and his full potential.

HARDY didn't let that napkin set him off course or distract him with negative feelings of self-doubt and discouragement. He released hit songs as a country artist and built a loyal audience that became obsessed with him and his music. His fans were die-hard. But what happened next was a testament to how strongly HARDY believes in himself and his vision. The release of *The Mockingbird & the Crow* is one of the best evolutionary transitions I've ever seen from an artist. The album admitted that he spent the first part of his career playing country music because that's what the people wanted to hear. The crowd, the radio producers, and the labels wanted country, so HARDY gave them country. But this album was an opportunity to write, record, and perform the music he wanted to play, which was rock music, so a rock album is what he released.

HARDY experienced doubt that night in 2015 when he picked up the napkin with "quit" written across it. He persevered. He then experienced doubt when he made the decision to leave the country music scene and pursue rock. He stayed focused on what he wanted to do and ignored the doubters. Through both scenarios, and I'm sure many more, he succeeded. His relentless drive to follow his ambitions and build the life he wanted—one inspired by his passions and what he believed in—led him to greatness. If at any point in that journey he would have stopped building because others doubted him, he would have never, ever climbed to where he is today.

Other people will call you crazy. They will doubt your

journey, choices, goals, and desires. That's okay. Let them doubt you. Let them root against you. As long as what you are doing is legal, moral, ethical, and right by the word of God, not one person can tell you otherwise. Everyone can doubt you. But until you start doubting yourself, none of that matters. That doubt can't influence your drive, motivation, or discipline to achieve greatness. Don't let that doubt break you because doubt is only dangerous when you start doubting yourself. Watching others work toward the life they dream of, despite the negativity around them from people rooting in the opposite direction, inspires me beyond belief. It is so beautiful when someone is confident in what they want to do and what brings them joy, and they aren't afraid to be unapologetically themselves.

Chapter Eight

LEGACY CAN'T BE BOUGHT. IT MUST BE BUILT.

"An authentic path may take longer, but the
moves and impact are forever legendary."
—Unknown

All of us are writing the story of our lives. Every decision and indecision creates ripples in that story, which have the potential to shift our trajectory forever. Sometimes if we're fortunate, we get to see the impact our story has on others.

Ashton Kutcher starred as the main character in *The Butterfly Effect*, which premiered in 2004. This movie is about a college student named Evan Treborn who suffers from painful headaches that cause frequent blackouts. During these moments of unconsciousness, Evan is able to travel back in time and relive moments of his childhood. Not only is he able to re-experience the past, but he is also able to alter the decisions he made and actions he took to drastically change the future. While this may seem like he discovered a way to cheat the system and create the dream life he always wanted, the opposite was true. While making some situations better, he also made other situations worse—much worse. He learned how some of the smallest changes to his past could completely alter the outcome of his future. That is the power of our choices and actions. They have a monumental impact on how we live, where we end up, and the legacy we leave behind even after we are gone.

There are many other books, movies, and stories that demonstrate the consequences of time travel (as if it were a reality), but *The Butterfly Effect* is one that left an impact on me. The trauma Evan experienced and created for other people in his life was so profound that the results were unfixable. The smallest changes to the decisions he made and the opportunities he pursued left him living a completely different life, one that was unrecognizable from his previous one. It made me realize the power of our decisions and how they impact our lives, the people around us, and the legacies we leave after we are gone.

The Ten-Year Mark

August of 2022 was a pivotal month in my life. I was in the thick of a life transition as a new dad and trying to navigate my new responsibilities as we were celebrating ten years in business. One decade before, I was sitting in my small college apartment in Indiana, Pennsylvania, registering my business with the state and starting my journey as an entrepreneur. What I believed I was capable of accomplishing just ten years prior was a fraction of where I like to imagine my potential exists today. To celebrate our ten-year anniversary, my team and I decided to activate the BPN community and show our gratitude for all the support our customers had shown us over the years. So we hosted an event in Austin, Texas. We invited friends, family, fans, and customers of the brand. People flew in from all over the country, and some even traveled internationally to join us. We logged some miles downtown, opened a pop-up shop in a small home in East Austin, and hosted a meet and greet with our community. Before we kicked off the run, with energy at an all-time high, a woman walked up to me with her seven-year-old daughter.

"I just want to thank you," she told me. The woman proceeded to tell me that her daughter didn't have a male father figure in the household, so she showed her daughter the content I created and the message I shared. I was that male role model for her daughter.

For a moment, I just stood there, taken aback.

Over the years, I had heard so many remarkable stories about how I helped people take control of their life and reach their fitness goals. I had seen how applying the Go One More mindset transformed them. Those stories are, and will always be, powerful, but hearing this woman's story was different. Maybe it was because I was a new dad to a beautiful baby girl, but it was very powerful to hear this mother tell me her story. I felt impacted and inspired in a way I had never felt before. And I still think about that conversation frequently. That conversation became a part of my North Star. It became a significant part of my meaningful mission.

My eyes were opened that day. I could see firsthand the real impact my story and content were making and the responsibility that came with that. This was the legacy I was building. This is the legacy I need to continue working toward. This is why I do what I do and why I must continue doing what I've been doing since I started. That day changed my life.

You know when someone asks you to take a photo of them and a group of friends? It could be a familiar face or a stranger that is passing by. If you're like me, as they hand their phone off to you, the first thing you do is grab the corner of your shirt and wipe off the camera lenses so the image turns out as crisp and clear as possible. What you did there was create an opportunity of clarity for that photo, which may end up becoming a significant memory for those people. That is exactly what that woman did for me that day. She provided me with clarity that left a lasting impression and shaped my perspective on the legacy I'm responsible for building.

Your story comes down to the collection of meaningful missions you choose to pursue during your lifetime. Your North Star determines how those meaningful missions fit the context of your purpose and the legacy you leave behind.

Legacy is really important to me, and I believe a lot of people get it wrong. They think that legacy is just what people say about you when you are dead: "He was extremely generous." "He was so humble." "He was an amazing entre-preneur." "He was a great athlete." "He made a lot of money." "He lived in a big house." For some people, this is enough, but for me, it's not.

Legacy for me is much larger. It changes the lives of the people you have impacted because it guides the way they think and act—forever. This is why as I transition into this next chapter of life, being a role model is at the forefront of my priorities. You won't be a role model for everyone, but you can be one for those whose values and beliefs are aligned with yours. I want to encourage you to think about your own legacy and how to strengthen it. A legacy is built from the choices we make for our meaningful mission, the ownership we accept with the decisions we pursue, the actions we take, and the courage we display.

Purpose and Direction

It's no surprise that anyone who has ever accomplished any-thing had to, at some point, just start. But where do you start? What should you focus your time on, and how do you get started in the first place? I love the story Bedros Keuil-ian shared with me about the need for purpose in our lives. While he was on my podcast, he told a great story about a dog named Cookie they got when his kids were younger. Cookie was part Mastiff, part German Shepherd, and even though she was only eight months old when they got her, she was a big dog. Shortly after they brought Cookie home, she began digging holes all over the yard and destroying their entire property. So Bedros decided to bring a trainer in to help them. After spending several weeks with Cookie, the dog trainer told him that he needed to give this type of dog a clear purpose, direction, and mission. These dogs are highly active animals, and in the absence of purpose and direction from their owners, they will create their own. And because Cookie was not given a clear purpose and direction from the beginning, she created her own ... digging holes all over Bedros's yard.

Holy shit, Bedros thought. *This is just like us.*

"That's humans, all of us," he told me. "Every single one of us, myself included. In the absence of service, routine, structure, and purpose, I will dig holes in my life. I will self-destruct."

That illustration reinforced a belief of mine that if I ever start self-destructing or self-sabotaging my life (which I've done before, still do from time to time, and will probably end up doing again in the future), it's because I'm not very clear on my meaningful mission at that period of time. I have to be proactive, take a step back, and make intentional decisions that reinforce what it is that I'm meant to be working on. We have to constantly assess how we show up for our responsibilities and serve them properly. Because if we don't, we will begin digging holes in the key areas of our lives that require careful attention.

So what did Bedros's dog Cookie teach me? First off, in the absence of purpose and direction, we will oftentimes provide ourselves with a mission that is self-destructive and lacks meaning. But more importantly, the issues that we might be experiencing from the day-to-day cannot be solved with a quick-flexed reaction, a verbal command, or simple acknowledgement. A foundation must be laid and built upon. The solution to feeling lost, confused, and self-destructive is the foundation of purpose, direction, and meaningful mission.

Arthur Brooks, the author of *From Strength to Strength*, teaches a very popular class at Harvard University on happiness. He explains that there are four factors that contribute to our happiness: faith, family, community, and meaningful work. I believe happiness and legacy are more closely associated than we often think or want to believe.

Can we build a legacy that we are truly proud of if we sacrifice happiness to achieve it? Or does that make us an imposter, a fake, a phony, or a critic? Here, I want to focus on one of those four factors and how it contributes to our purpose: faith.

One of the reasons I fell in love with the concept of having a meaningful mission is because it is adaptable and changes based on the seasons of life, responsibilities, and goals. Purpose can feel lofty, especially when we talk about it in the absence of faith. Brooks says that "faith is anything transcendent that helps you escape the boring sitcom that your life is." He also says that "you need relief, you need perspective, and you need peace. The only way to do that is to get little. It is to get small. And the way to do that is to zoom out. You have to zoom out of your life. That is transcendence. And you have to practice it every day."

Perspective on its own can change your entire outlook on life in a matter of seconds; it did for me in June of 2019. My mom was diagnosed with ovarian cancer just six months prior, and sooner than we realized, we were sitting at home in her last few days alive on hospice care. The day before she passed away, my brother and I sat next to her bed and she told us, "If you ever want to see me again, you have to believe in God."

In that moment, I zoomed out of my life. Everything I thought mattered didn't matter any longer. I realized my mom wasn't going to experience the next couple chapters with me. She was going to miss my wedding, the birth of my children, and the many life experiences after that. It put life into perspective. I wanted to see her again, so from that moment on, I committed to building a relationship with the Lord.

Now, for me, faith is my relationship with God as a Christian and as a believer in Jesus Christ. You may or may not share those same beliefs as me, but I am confident that my purpose is to be a servant of God and obedient in His word. I'm not perfect by any means, and it is constant work, but that faith and belief is the foundation of my purpose.

I don't believe that our purpose is our work, but I do believe we can fulfill our purpose *through* our work. While our purpose remains the foundation, steadfast and strong, our meaningful mission can evolve, adapt, and change. So how do you apply this? Think about laying the foundation. What is your purpose? How do you practice your faith? What do you believe in? From there, fulfill that purpose through your meaningful mission and work. There will be periods of time where that meaningful mission is fuzzy, unclear, or empty, but that is your opportunity to sharpen the axe in preparation for your next season. If you stay true to your purpose and intentionally fulfill it through your work toward your

North Star, you will be on the path of building a legacy you can stand behind—something you are proud of and that represents your values and beliefs. It will be authentically you.

Legacy Requires Ownership

Look at your life today. Who and what do you see? Where you are, who you're with, and what you're doing is the sum of all the decisions you've made in the past years. The good and bad, the wins and losses, the successes and failures all account for and contribute to this result. You have to own where you are at any point in your life. It doesn't matter if you're twenty, forty, sixty, or eighty years old. It is a personal responsibility to own that.

If you're not where you want to be, you can't blame anyone else. You can't blame the economy. You can't blame your family. You can't blame your friends. You can't blame your boss or your job. There needs to be an act of ownership and accountability. Jocko Willink and Leif Babin wrote an incredible book titled *Extreme Ownership* on this entire concept. They said, "Once people stop making excuses, stop blaming others, and take ownership of everything in their lives, they are compelled to take action to solve their problems. They are better leaders, better followers, more dependable and actively contributing team members, and more skilled in aggressively driving toward mission accomplishment." It must be part of your mission to take ownership of the choices you are faced with and the outcomes you experience that lead to the life you live.

In order to accomplish goals and find success, we must choose to grow. And it doesn't happen independently or overnight. Growth doesn't happen on its own. We must wake up and choose growth, day in and day out. Growth isn't free from failure or mistakes. It usually invites them. And if we are being honest, most growth is the direct result of more bad than good. This isn't to say that you should pursue poor choices, but don't be afraid of them through the pursuit of greatness.

I imagine the day before I pass, as I'm on my death bed, will be the most honest day of my life. I will be at peace. I will be able to look back at all the seasons and choices I've lived and decided. At that point, I will have truly tapped my potential. Full potential? Maybe. I hope so. But there won't be any more days of discovery. The journey, which I love so much, will have reached its final chapter, and I will have no other choice but to own where I am, the relationships I've maintained, and the things I've accomplished. We can't blame others for what went wrong or what misguided the trajectory of our life. Where we end up is the sum of the millions upon millions of decisions we made up until that point—the big ones that felt monumental and the small ones that seemed insignificant. When that day comes, I want to be proud of the man I've become and the legacy I've built.

Built in Drops and Lost in Buckets

The beautiful thing about legacy is that it has to be built. It can't be bought, sold, or cheated. There are no shortcuts, fast tracks, or express lanes to building a true legacy that you can be proud of. The building process requires endurance, brick by brick, just like a mason lays the foundation and erects the walls, one brick at a time, over and over again until a house forms and a home is established. As I'm sure you are aware at this point in the book, nothing great comes fast or easy, and if it does, it is probably too good to be true. Be cautious of these catchy opportunities that may present themselves to you throughout your lifetime.

I like to think of the legacy that I am intentionally building as a bucket. You begin your life with an empty bucket. It is free from dirt, cracks, erosion, and debris. It is shiny, colorful, and pristine. That bucket is sitting below a faucet, and it is ready to be filled with whatever you decide to fill it with. Now, you can turn that faucet on full blast if you desire. This will fill up your bucket the fastest, but you won't be able to control what goes in. The water moves so quickly that you'll have no time to monitor the quality of the water that enters. This is how many people approach their lives, and by the time they reach their final days on earth, they wonder how they got to where they are today. Where did they go wrong? Well, it's hard to say because they didn't control the choices, decisions, or actions that led them to the legacy they created. It was fast-paced, careless, unintentional, and reckless. We often think of legacy as this proud, monumental statue of the life we created that is praised for all the good things we accomplished. For some, this is true. But for others, the opposite may be the reality.

This bucket that we have the responsibility of filling is our legacy. Instead of trying to build a legacy with speed and agility, let's try and slow down. Be deliberate. Be intentional. Make decisions with the clarity they require to guide us in the appropriate direction. Filling the bucket in this way will most definitely take longer. Go ahead and turn that faucet so the water slowly comes to a drip. One drop at a time. If at any point the water quality decreases, becomes contaminated, or the bucket needs repair, we can make the necessary changes to the flow and fill. That is how we build a legacy we will be proud of. Slowly. Intentionally. Carefully. Drop by drop. Brick by brick.

As a young entrepreneur growing up in a competitive industry, I was fortunate to be mentored by some great people along the way. Some of them I talked to daily, and some I never talked with personally. Instead, I read their books, listened to their podcasts, and followed their stories. I study successful entrepreneurs, athletes, world leaders, and philosophers. We should be so incredibly grateful for how accessible life-changing content is in today's digital world, but yet so many people still don't take advantage of it. Those are the same individuals who fail to take ownership and responsibility for the outcomes of their lives. Kevin Plank, the founder and CEO of Under Armour said, "Brands are all about trust. That trust is built in drops and lost in buckets." I'll never forget that. Not only was it applicable to my entrepreneurial journey, but it's applicable to our entire lives. Our legacy.

You could spend a lifetime building your legacy, drop by drop, and ruin it overnight. There is no such thing as overnight success, but there is such a thing as overnight destruction and failure. After years and years of filling that bucket with intentional drops of water, it can easily be kicked over by the wrong choices and decisions. While this may intimidate many people from ever getting started in the first place, it should encourage you to maintain ownership and accountability. Just because you build a legacy doesn't mean it's bulletproof, indestructible, or free from failure. The bigger you build it, the tougher those choices become. The more people you involve, the harder it is to hold the standard. And the less responsibility you control, the more likely that bucket will tip over and empty across the ground.

In my opinion, where most people go wrong is that they stop following their intuition. They become distracted from their purpose, and they allow other people to dictate the trajectory of their life, story, and legacy. People will try to tell you what to do and how to do it. If you don't listen to them, they may become angry and resentful. You don't want those people in your life, but more importantly, you don't want to follow their advice. If you are a people pleaser, this will get you in trouble. People pleasing will lead you on a path that goes nowhere. And it is no way to build a legacy. Stay true to yourself, your values, and the decisions you make. It will significantly increase your chances of building the legacy you desire.

A Generational Inflection Point

It's a shame that so many people reach the end of their life and feel like they haven't experienced a full one. It's because of the family they were born into, where they were raised, a lack of resources, a lack of mentorship, low-paying jobs, and so on and so forth. (This goes back to my conversation with Bedros Keuilian that I shared in chapter 2.) What holds most people back from reaching their full potential? It's the story they tell themselves. The story of why they didn't and why they couldn't. These stories are full of blame and lack responsibility. This is not to say that people are not born into environments and situations that lack the things they need to succeed, but we have a choice to make a change. That choice is going to be uncomfortable, inconvenient, and difficult, but it's a choice we have the ability to make.

I'm not going to act like I was raised in a household, geographic location, or environment that was troubled. I had it pretty good. My family is from a small town in central Pennsylvania surrounded by rolling hills and beautiful farmland. My mom was a schoolteacher, and my dad worked as a programmer for businesses' computer information systems. My brother, who is three years younger, and I played team sports growing up, and our parents were at every game. We spent quality time with our extended family, went on vacations every year, and we were loved. My parents didn't start my business for me, but they were supportive. They didn't step in when things got hard, but they were a phone call away to listen to my struggles. To be honest, I had the childhood I dream my children will have, and I wish more kids around the world could experience it. But that isn't the case for everyone, and I acknowledge that.

With that being said, some of the most successful entrepreneurs, athletes, and world leaders have come from the complete opposite environment that I experienced as a child. They were born in a poor country, starved as they lived off scraps, couldn't find enough money to fund a proper education, and didn't have anyone else in their life that found a way to break the streak. How did they do it? Courage. They had the courage to make the executive decision for change.

Now, you may hear this and think, *Well, yeah, but those people are the exception to the rule. For most people, the life they are born into is the life they are stuck with.* And that is true. But who says you can't be the exception? Who says you can't be the 1 percent of people who make that big change? You can be the one person who breaks the streak in your family and becomes the one who marks the generational inflection point.

An inflection point marks a significant change. It is the point of a curve at which a change in direction occurs. We typically see trends in families, communities, and people in general. Occupation, income status, marital success, and levels of education are normally consistent within these populations. And we tend to accept the outcome of our life by what and who we are surrounded by. But the truth is you can be the generational inflection point in your family or society. The courage you demonstrate can initiate a change that shifts the trajectory of the legacy you leave and inspires generations to come. It's a personal responsibility to be that person for the generations that follow. It will not only change your life, but many others after you as well. That is impact. That is legacy.

A generational inflection point can change the course of your life, your family members' lives, and the lives of the generations that follow. You can be the first person who goes to college, you can be the first person who embraces a life of health and fitness, you can be the person who follows Jesus Christ, you can be the person who creates financial freedom. You can be the first person in your family history that does any and all of those things, even if no one before you has done it. To be that person, however, you will have to be courageous enough to take the first step, lead your family to a new way of life, and be the generational inflection point.

Being the generational inflection point doesn't mean you have to change the world. You don't have to be the next Jeff Bezos or Bill Gates. You might not run for president, discover the cure for cancer, or sell a business you bootstrapped for millions of dollars, but that's not necessarily the goal. The intent is to shift the trajectory of what you and your family believe is possible. It's having the courage to try and potentially fail. Sometimes people just need to see other people putting it all on the line, swing for the fences, and go all in on their goals to be inspired to try themselves.

I had a friend growing up who was raised in a household that was against everything healthy. His parents thought working out was a waste of time and eating a well-balanced, nutritious diet was too obsessive. Not only did his parents live this way, but so did his grandparents and his great grandparents. His extended family, including uncles, aunts, and cousins, also lived unhealthy lifestyles. They were all severely overweight, had high blood pressure and pre-diabetes, and were on a path of early death and disease.

When my friend graduated high school and started college with me, he decided he wanted to make a change. At first, it wasn't anything crazy. He wanted to start going to the gym and making smarter food choices. He wanted to get leaner and feel better. The more time he spent focused on his health and fitness, the better he felt. His energy levels increased, his sleep quality improved, his mood was significantly better, and his self-confidence transformed in a very positive way.

Instead of spending his time playing video games, going out to bars, eating pizza, and binge-watching Netflix, he was now dedicating all of his free time to becoming a learning machine. He began reading books on nutrition, watching workout videos on YouTube, and attending fitness expos on the weekends to connect with other people who had a shared passion. Eventually, he even changed his major from accounting to nutrition, with a focus on becoming a registered dietician.

My friend not only changed his life, but saved it, too. And in the process, he shifted the trajectory of his family's health and created a generational inflection point. His parents, uncles, aunts, cousins, and siblings all saw the positive impact he was making. At first, they were hesitant to join him, but eventually, they came around. They saw how much better he felt and how much better he looked. He shared with them the negative health consequences of the lifestyle they were living and how to make a change, so they did. Because of my friend's work, passion, and life-changing experience, he was able to improve the lives of both current and future family members, for generations to come. That is the power each one of us holds if we have the courage to make the choice.

If you want to build a legacy you are proud of that reaches your full potential, be resourceful. Pick up the book. Listen to the podcast. Read the article. Study those who have come before you. Maybe one day someone will be reading a book about the life you lived because you had the courage to be the one who reset the generational inflection point for your family and community.

The Lighthouse

We live in a very dark, negative, and noisy world. I feel this calling—this responsibility—to be a light in all of the noise and darkness. We should all feel this calling to shine a light on what is accepted but wrong. Call it out and initiate the change. When others try and pull you down, stand for what you believe in. Fight for your values and principles. Like Alexander Hamilton said, "Those who stand for nothing fall for anything."

This concept has always made me think of a lighthouse. The visual and functional representation of a lighthouse is to be a source of truth, a guiding light for those lost at sea, off course, and off mission. If you think of a lighthouse, it's a physical structure that is rooted in the ground. Its one job is to be a signal for ships and sailors. The darker it becomes, the more important the lighthouse's job. Waves crash upon its foundation and attempt to erode it away from the shoreline. Sea creatures attach to it, climb up it, and eat away at the material it was built from. A lighthouse takes a real brutal beating over time, but you can still find them standing after hundreds of years—through multiple generations, many storms, and equal amounts of dark and light. They are a shining light that says, "Follow me." This light is faithful. It is obedient. It is reliable. It is firm in its foundation. The waves, the erosion, the weather, and all sorts of people and animals will try to destroy this light, but it remains firm and strong. It provides direction and has a very intentional meaningful mission.

My mom, Linda Bare, was a lighthouse. In June of 2019, she passed away from cancer, but the legacy she left on this world and the people she reached was remarkable. She never had to tell my brother and me how to live a great life; she showed us. My mom was a selfless servant to her family, friends, work, and God. She spent her professional career and much of her personal life teaching special education and coaching Special Olympics. She was funny, joyful, energetic, passionate, caring, and spontaneous. Even when my mom's life got dark and she was deep in the throes of chemotherapy and aggressive pain medication, she still showed up as the lighthouse. She taught me how to be tough. She taught me how to be strong. She taught me how to be vulnerable and empathetic. She taught me everything I needed to know about building a legacy that I could be proud of.

I feel this responsibility to be a light in the darkness. That is the legacy I want to leave. To me, that means being a role model. I feel this responsibility as a father, as a leader, as a business owner, as a friend, and as a content creator. Every piece of content I share, whether audio, video, or still, is part of my story. The story we are writing has the ability to change many lives, not just our own. So write that story wisely because it can change the world.

Chapter Nine

YOU CAN GO FAST ALONE, BUT YOU CAN GO MUCH FURTHER TOGETHER

"The people who are crazy enough to think they can change the world are the ones who do."

—Steve Jobs

f we compare our lives to a footrace, it can be measured in miles. Let's say, hypothetically, we all live to one hundred years old. One of the most common and sought after distances for people crazy enough to sign up for an ultra-marathon is one hundred miles. In a one-hundred-mile race, anything can happen, many things can go wrong, but significant acts of greatness can be achieved, too. The race is more than the miles. The race is an experience that can't be truly explained by just units of linear measurement; there is so much more to it. There are highs and lows, injuries, trips and falls, deep conversations, and lonely moments. There is banter with your crew early on and conversations with God late into the night.

Like I mentioned in the beginning of this book, these races for me are no longer for a notch on my belt or a medal to hang. These races need to unlock a part of me that hasn't been explored before. There needs to be a deeper discovery with these big efforts. And one of the biggest unlocks I've discovered when it comes to these efforts (races and life) is that you can go fast alone, but you can go much further together.

It's not just traveling *with* others, but the results that come from it. When we have the right people, who are aligned with our values and mission, fighting alongside us, the possibilities are up to our imaginations. The right people will support us, push us, and hold us accountable to do more. I once believed that traveling with others would slow me down, and sometimes it does, but the distance you can travel together is much further. Life is more than the miles. It's the quality of the distance and the people who travel with us.

"The Lone Wolf" Lie

American author and blogger Mark Manson once said, "If you cringe at your former self, that's good—it means you've grown. Never stop cringing."

Before the BPN team and community existed, it used to be just me, and I considered myself a lone wolf. I was proud of it. I bragged about it. Now, just as Manson explained, I cringe at it. Being an entrepreneur can be a lonely life. That's just the reality of it; it's a life that not everybody is cut out to pursue. In the beginning, I was naïve, bootstrapped, and in way over my head. But you don't know what you don't know. I had no demand for the product I was selling, and no one knew what Bare Performance Nutrition was or what BPN even stood for. So, I operated very quickly and oftentimes very alone. That's what I did because that is what I had to do. Over the years, I've learned that yes, you can go fast alone, but you can go much further together.

I used to take a lot of pride in doing things solo. It made me feel accomplished, providing me with the responsibility of success or failure and granting me complete control. I didn't have to rely on anyone else. I thought I didn't need anyone else. There was no one to disappoint me, and I could streamline every process. But that only worked for a period of time, and as BPN grew, that mindset held me back.

Now, don't get me wrong, I still believe most "startups" need this season. There aren't many other ways around it, but knowing that it might not last forever is important. Very important. And understanding how to transition from a solo mission to a team journey is exciting yet challenging. Whether you are building a business or working toward a personal goal, there will be many times when you need to operate solo. These lessons aren't an excuse to not get started now because you don't have a team to support you. Rather, they are to reinforce that we can do much more when we work together, collaboratively, not independently.

A few years after getting the brand off the ground and generating some sales, my brother Preston joined me. He was the first person who really believed in me and took a massive risk by joining me and contributing to my vision. Eventually, my vision also became his vision, and we have been building together since he made the move to Texas in 2016.

Now, a comment that I see frequently and a message that I receive almost daily is "How do I find my people?"

If you are true to what you believe in and firm on the values you stand upon, then they will find you. And you will find them. You're not going to do it by sitting in your home or surfing the web. You're not going to do it with an exclusively digital connection, either. You're going to have to put yourself out there. If that is uncomfortable, which it is for many, I encourage you to embrace that discomfort. Find places, events, and activations that resonate with your meaningful mission. If they don't exist, create them. Maybe that in itself is your meaningful mission. Have the courage to place yourself in situations that create the opportunities you desire.

But like I previously stated, I still believe most "startups" need a season of solo building. This may be weeks, months, or even years. There are businesses, projects, and missions that I'm working on today that are still being done alone, but if that was the case for everything I do, I would be quite lonely. Minimizing the number of people involved in certain parts of the building process is critical. It allows you to maintain focus, clearly build your foundation, and create values that are essential to you and your future. Don't resist or fear starting or building by yourself, but be careful of viewing yourself as a lone wolf.

In the early days of creating content, filming videos, and sharing my life with the world, I started to become self-conscious of my older work. It was embarrassing, and I was tempted to delete older things I created to paint myself in a more professional and polished light. I'm glad I didn't because, at the time, I was sharing my passions and work in the most authentic way possible.

We are never going to start something meaningful with all the answers. The path from where you are now to where you want to be may be blurry. You will do things, say things, and think things that you cringe at years later, but that's okay. That is growth. Be proud of that growth. I now go back and watch or read previous pieces I published to remind myself of how far I've come and how much I've grown. The old stuff is gold. It's the treasure that makes the legacy you are building that much sweeter, not just for yourself, but for others who are struggling with the journey as well. It's all part of the process. Embrace it. I once had a chip on my shoulder. I set out to prove everyone wrong who didn't believe in me or support my dreams and aspirations. I thought the most efficient way from point A to point B was the most effective way: alone.

In all reality, it was just a few short years ago when I

internally referred to myself as a lone wolf. No one understood me and what I was trying to accomplish. Everyone around me was thinking too small, while I was thinking *big*. I would say things like, "You're either with me or against me." My perspective was small because my experience was limited. I also believed in this "lone wolf" lie because it was being promoted by influential entrepreneurs online. They sure fooled me.

Some things you have to learn the hard way. But I was all about hard. I thrived in it. In the thick of building the business, I just kept going. *I don't need friends. I don't need family. I understand what I'm trying to do and what I'm building.*

Sometimes when I look back at my younger self, I have to laugh. *Nick, you had no clue. You didn't know what the hell you were saying.* I look at life in a completely different way now. Becoming a father changed me, but my view shifted even before my kids were born. There is no doubt about it; I love building. I've always loved building. I'm obsessed with building BPN, building the life I desire for my family, building meaningful relationships, building my fitness and my body. But I don't want to build alone anymore. I want to build with my community, with people who share the same values and beliefs that I do. I don't want to go on this journey alone anymore because the impact we can create in the world is much stronger when there is a force behind it, not just a person.

I came to realize that doing anything great alone is not going to provide you with the outcome you're expecting. The journey is much more than the miles you have traveled.

Living a life of Go One More isn't always what you have accomplished, but how you have accomplished it and who you
have accomplished it with.

More Than the Miles

I had heard about the Leadville 100 for years. Everybody
would talk about this legendary, mythical ultramarathon in
the Rocky Mountains of Leadville, Colorado—fifty miles out
and fifty miles back, ascending and descending 15,600 feet.
As I shared earlier, my lottery ticket was pulled in 2021, giving me the opportunity to run the trail. But I wasn't running
it alone. At this point in BPN history, I had amazing people surrounding me who were always quick to jump in, offer
solutions, and help. So we all went to Leadville, Colorado, to
compete as a team and document our experience. We embodied the theme of "If You Want to Go Fast, Go Alone, but
If You Want to Go Far, Go Together."

Simply calling this a one-hundred-mile race doesn't give
it the justice it deserves. There are many factors that compound and come together—the team, the crews, the support—to make this race possible. So I wasn't the only one
racing. It was the entire BPN team doing Leadville 100 together. While I was the only person physically running the
one-hundred-mile course, the crew contributed just as much,
if not more. A solid crew can make or break your ultra. You
need a committed team. They will carry and prepare some of
your fuel sources at checkpoints, help you refill anything you

have run out of, and support you through some of the most challenging points of the race. (You can see the truth of this in BPN's documentary *More Than the Miles*.)

The moment we landed in Leadville, we all started working together to prepare for the big day. We drove to the checkpoints, scouted locations, inspected the terrain and routes, familiarized everyone with the map, and conducted rehearsals/walk-throughs for different parts of the race. The night before the Leadville 100 started, we had a team meeting where we walked through each phase of the race, broken down by checkpoints. Everyone had maps and documents that laid out my plan, an ETA for each checkpoint, and the nutrition/equipment I would require to pick up/leave at specific locations. By the time the race started, everyone in the crew knew their role, responsibilities, and the plan.

One of the things I loved about being in the military and the infantry was that there was this camaraderie I had never found anywhere else before. We had built that same thing within BPN. The person to the left of you and the right of you wanted to see you succeed. They wanted to help you win. They wanted to help you get there. It wasn't an "I" or "me"; it was a "we," a team thing. Each person played such a vital role and was 100 percent committed to the mission of our organization. Our mindset was that we were willing to do whatever it took to accomplish this goal. When you surround yourself with the right people in your life, they will take that responsibility and accountability, and they will hold some of that so you don't have to hold it all (even when you feel like you are).

The race was hard. There was a time that I reached a point where my whole world began to close up and things went dark. But that is why you sign up for hard things like this in the first place. You want to feel and experience those dark places. It's through those extremes that you find things out about yourself. You discover strengths and weaknesses that you never would have found unless you did it.

By the time we got to the base of what was the finish line, the entire BPN team was there. Everybody began to run with me, and we crossed the finish line together, completing this dream we started together. Everyone knew and realized that they had a massive role in this accomplishment that we achieved together. It's one of the moments I will always remember because of the journey it took to get there. It's a clear example of the power that exists when people come together.

It's an incredible thing to find people who are committed to something greater than yourself because when you accomplish things together, it is truly fulfilling. Leadville 100 proved this truth in life: If you want to go fast, go alone. But if you want to go far, go together.

"Two years ago, there were four of us," Stef said when talking about the Leadville 100. "Now, there's all these people who are all in on Nick's crazy dream. And it's not just Nick's dream anymore. It's all of our crazy dream."

You Need the Right People

A few years ago, Ben Francis, cofounder and CEO of Gymshark, visited the BPN headquarters with a few members of his team. He was conducting some business in Texas and carved out a day to catch up and go out for dinner. Ben has built an impressive brand and organization. Impressive doesn't even do it justice. It's incredible. Remarkable. I resonated with his story as I watched Gymshark become the company it is today while I was sitting in my college apartment building BPN. I first saw Gymshark enter the fitness scene when a few young YouTubers started wearing the apparel, and before I knew it, Gymshark was everywhere. Their apparel can be found on at least one person in every gym you walk into. He had a vision, and he went for it. All in.

As Ben and I walked around the BPN warehouse, he told me something I'll never forget. He said, "There are three things that determine the success or failure of a business: people, brand, and product." You need all three if you want to win in this space. You need the best product, the best brand, and, of course, the best people. People build businesses, and you will never go far with the wrong people on your team or in your life.

In his book *For the Culture*, Marcus Collins says there is a system that explains the characteristics of a culture (or a brand). System one is how we see the world. "Understanding who we are is a fundamental human drive," Collins said, "This designation, our identity, acts as a compass that guides how we see the world . . . the second system of culture is a shared way of life. This refers to the way a group of people behave and live in accordance with their shared beliefs and ideologies."

We naturally are attracted to individuals and groups of people who see the world as we do and share the same beliefs and ideologies. It's that simple. This makes building relationships easier, with much less resistance. It leads to more collaboration, stronger communities, and a more fulfilling life.

When I first started BPN, I had to operate as a lone wolf. It was my only choice, and it worked at the time. People ask me all the time how I built the team we have today. The truth is, the team kind of built itself. From the beginning, I was very vocal and persistent about who BPN was, the mission we served, and the values that represented the foundation of what we were to build upon. I shared these things loudly and frequently in person, at events, and through my content. I even tattooed "Go One More" on my arm in 2019. Since then, thousands of others have done the same. By sharing my personal beliefs and worldview, I attracted a culture and created a community. It's been powerful, one of the most powerful forces I've ever experienced. It's a type of power and level of energy that you can feel in its presence. Through this network and community, I organically came across the right people, at the right time, to join BPN. Building the team in those first couple of years wasn't that hard, if I'm being honest. I kept leaning into what I believed in, and more of the right people started showing up, raising their hands, and joining the movement.

When our team traveled to Leadville, Colorado, in 2021, we were shooting a documentary and communicating the idea that you can go fast alone, but you can go much further together. And I believed every word of that. But as the team grew and as the business evolved, I experienced the growing pains of a scaling organization. Something about that phrase didn't feel quite right anymore based on what I was learning as a business leader and founder. There had to be something added to the end of that statement, and I learned that the right words are "if you have the right people with you."

What sparked the caveat? Well, I became complacent. I let my guard down. I stopped trusting my gut. And I made decisions that lacked due diligence, intentionality, and discipline. I attracted the wrong people because my North Star became blurry and my vision was no longer being vocalized. I stopped being the leader I needed to be for the people who made the choice to join our community. We hired individuals who didn't share our values or believe in the mission. Other team members failed to grow with the business or lost passion for their work, and we kept them on the team longer than we should have. It wasn't good for either party and resulted in anger, resentment, and an unhealthy culture.

My decision to step down from the CEO role of BPN, move to Nashville, and step out of an operational role in the business had negative consequences. When I made all these decisions, they felt like the right ones, but I ultimately realized that they were not. I learned from these choices. Not immediately, but eventually, they caught up to me. In Colin Powell's memoir, *My American Journey*, he said, "Leadership is solving problems. The day soldiers stop bringing you their problems is the day you have stopped leading them. They have either lost confidence that you can help or concluded you do not care. Either case is a failure of leadership." At this point, the team, our community, and the culture didn't have all the right people, and it was driving us in an unwanted direction. While we still had strong individuals who contributed to the team, believed in the mission, and shared my beliefs, they stopped bringing me their problems. I had stopped leading them.

Having the wrong people on your team, in your business, or just in your life is like a poison. Eventually, these poisons spread so fast and far that they can cause severe damage, illness, or death. The same happens when you have the wrong people on board. For lack of a better term, they are a poison. They are invited into your ecosystem and slowly start attacking everything and everyone. The poison spreads to different parts of your life and departments. Eventually, it takes over everything. Everyone is affected.

If you have the wrong people with you, I'm sorry to tell you, but you can only go so far, and you definitely won't be able to reach your full potential. Those people will hold you back. They will limit how high the ceiling is but will lower the floor with every passing day. It's your personal responsibility as a leader—a leader of your life, a leader of your family, a leader of your business—to hold the standard for those who join your community. The best communities in the world are not necessarily the biggest, but they are the strongest. These communities understand the vision and shared beliefs that bring everyone together. You can go fast alone, but you can go much further together . . . if you have the right people.

Choose Allies over Enemies

As I think back to when I believed in "The Lone Wolf" lie, I realize I was immature and inexperienced. I lacked perspective and was naïve and insecure. I felt challenged by other people working toward similar goals as I was. I watched competitors, and even friends, building businesses and accomplishing their goals, and I became angry. I was resentful. I started to despise them and eventually viewed them as enemies. It was a horrible place to operate from, and it was an unhealthy approach to building my business and life. I wasn't being the leader or role model I wanted to be. It certainly wasn't Christlike.

Over the years, my mindset has shifted. People will become enemies if you view them as enemies, but they will also become allies if you view them as such. Just because someone is doing well in life, and maybe pursuing something very similar to you, doesn't mean it takes away from your potential. And instead of working against one another, in many cases, we can come together and accomplish more as a combined force. Just like former US President John F. Kennedy said, "A rising tide lifts all boats."

While this doesn't necessarily mean we need to partner with our competitors or join forces with our opponents, there are opportunities to choose an alliance instead of a war. In the introduction, I mentioned that one of my favorite podcasts is *Founders* by David Senra. In one of his episodes (#358), he discussed what he learned by spending some time with John Mackey, the cofounder of Whole Foods Market. Before Whole Foods was the massive natural food market it is today, it was just one store in Austin, Texas, operating out of a three-story house.

Mackey shared that in the early days of bootstrapping Whole Foods, wholesale pricing was tough. The grocery stores that had multiple locations received better pricing from the large distributors because they were purchasing at higher volumes, but because John just had one store, pricing was higher and margins were small. So, Whole Foods partnered with a few other natural food competitor stores so they could purchase in larger volumes and receive better pricing.

For some, that's a hard pill to swallow. Partner with your competitors? That's nonsense. But it worked, and all boats were lifted in the process.

The moral of that story is that we can go fast alone, but we can go much further together. I once viewed everyone who wasn't directly on my team as an enemy, and through that mindset, they did become an enemy. I've since accepted the fact that they don't need to be my enemy, and that by making them an ally, we can all win together. This shift transformed my relationships, approach to business, and happiness. I now feel more confident in leading a team and in the values I was instilling in them.

Call On the Coach

The goal of this book is to improve your clarity in life so you can Go One More in all things you do. Go One More is not only an action, but more importantly, it's an outcome. Sometimes we can't do that alone, and we need a coach to help us go from being all consumed to all in. I've hired coaches, asked for help, and sought out guidance many times in my life. And it's always been the right decision. Whether this person is someone you pay for their services or someone you trust for their honesty, you need someone in your corner. Someone who will tell you what you need to hear, not what you want to hear. The journey of life, especially when you are an ambitious individual, can be lonely and challenging.

People are everything. They bring us joy and they bring us sadness. They bring us hope and also hopelessness. They teach us love and they teach us evil. Some of the most important decisions we can make in our lives revolve around the people we choose to include in ours. Not only the people we spend our free time with, but also the people we work with, live with, listen to, and are coached by.

Coaches come in all shapes and sizes (literally and figuratively). I grew up playing team sports. I played baseball and ice hockey for most of my childhood, soccer for a few years, and football for a couple of seasons. I had dozens of head coaches and assistant coaches. A few stand out, but many of them blend in with the rest. That is nothing against them personally, but it's the reality. We would get super excited when an ex-pro athlete or former alumni record holder would come back to our small hometown of Palmyra, Pennsylvania, to coach us. I remember always thinking that, because of their track record and God-given talent for the game, they would turn us into state champs. It never happened. That's because the best coaches don't have to be the best athletes. They love the game and the athletes, but more importantly, they love to coach.

We interact with very good people, teams, ideas, and products on a daily basis. It's not uncommon to leave those moments feeling satisfied and happy, but the distance between very good and remarkable is significant. You leave a remarkable experience with memories you can't forget. A great coach, mentor, and guide will help you get from point A to point B, but a remarkable coach leaves an impact that changes the trajectory of your life and the success you achieve. A coach doesn't have to be someone who is running plays off the sidelines of a football field or someone who tells you if you are good enough to play on the varsity team. A remarkable coach is someone who you trust, someone who cares about your success, and someone whose guidance can help you Go One More in certain areas of your life.

Ryan Holiday is the author of many great books. In one of my favorites, *Ego Is the Enemy*, he says, "Ego is the enemy of what you want and of what you have: Of mastering a craft. Of real creative insight. Of working well with others. Of building loyalty and support. Of longevity. Of repeating and retaining your success. It repulses advantages and opportunities. It's a magnet for enemies and errors."

There is an ego associated with accomplishing things on your own, reaching success in the absence of others. I used to carry a lot of pride behind the fact that I didn't want or need help from anyone else. I thought I had all the answers and that partners, mentors, coaches, and guides would hold me back. The reality is I was afraid of the truth, which was that I didn't know what I was doing. My naïve and ignorant self didn't want to be told what I didn't know, so the only way to get where I wanted to be was alone. That ego held me back for many years. Don't get me wrong, I still made progress. But it wasn't the progress I could have made if I had asked for and accepted the help of others.

A coach doesn't have to be someone who is assigned to you or that you pay on a monthly basis for a few hours each week. Some of the best mentors I've had in my life helped me because they saw my potential and wanted to help me fulfill it. On the flip side, some of the best mentors I've had in my life cost me a lot. Some of the worst mentors cost me a lot, too, more than I could afford, but I had to learn that the hard way. Not everyone has the best intentions, and unfortunately, there is no way to know what incentivizes people and what behaviors they will exhibit to get what they want.

Jeff Cunningham is an example of a remarkable coach. He guided me from a 3:24 marathon to a 2:39 marathon in three years. Jeff woke up early and drove an hour from his home and family to coach me during training sessions. He flew across country in the middle of the night to congratulate me at the finish line of races. He picked up the phone every time I called, regardless of where he was or the time of day. Chris Hickey is another example of a remarkable mentor. Chris was the previous CEO of a popular sports nutrition brand, led multiple companies to successful exits, and guided founders and many consumer brands to strategic growth. Chris has been an advisor to me and BPN, which has led to one of the most meaningful professional relationships I have built over the years.

I've experienced remarkable coaches and horrible coaches. Some have helped me succeed, and others have helped themselves get ahead. A great partnership between a mentor and mentee is one where both parties win. The best coaches and mentors I've worked with, like Jeff and Chris, have led me in a direction of where I needed to go, not necessarily where I wanted to go. They have had the hard conversations with me. They have called me out on my bullshit (tactfully). They have recognized when I was all consumed by the process and pulled me out of it. They have made calls and decisions that may negatively affect their results, monetary gain, or timeline because it is in my best interest. Remarkable coaches and mentors exist, and I encourage you to find them. Sometimes they end up in your life by what feels like the grace of God, and other times, you have to work hard to seek them out. You can go fast alone, but you can go so much further together. But only when you have the right people with you.

Ready to find your remarkable coach? Here is a checklist to guide your search:

A remarkable coach or mentor should:

- Be someone you know—or can comfortably get to know—and trust
- Be someone you get along with and enjoy spending a lot of time with
- Be open and honest
- Be knowledgeable about your field or goal
- Make time for you when you need them (within reason)
- Share your values—at least the big ones
- Lead you to where you need to go, not necessarily where you want to go

- Show that they are dedicated and emotionally invested in your success
- Believe in you and push you toward uncomfortable limits

Be careful who you take advice from, but at the end of the day, trust your gut.

The Manifesto

In December of 2023, I shared the following manifesto with all the employees of BPN. A few days after sharing it with the team, I shared it on social media. I drafted this manifesto late one night when I couldn't sleep. It was around the same time I had decided to move back to Texas, close down the Nashville office, and reassume the CEO position. This was more than a set of motivational sentences; it was the vision for the future of my company and a promise to everyone involved.

> 2024 is going to be different. This is the year we show up as our true, authentic, unapologetic selves. It's how BPN started, and it's how we were built. You can't buy brand story, mission, or vision. It has to be created. It's forged through hardship. It's born by toughness.
>
> We fuel performance. We fuel individuals through training, supplements, nutrition, education, content, motivation, and by showing them how to be tough.

Real toughness is not for show. It's not intended to intimidate. It is the ability to pursue greatness without sacrifice of integrity. It is choosing the hard right over the easy wrong. Toughness is a driven commitment through confidence.

We have changed lives—transformed from rock bottom. That is the power of going more. It has saved people from their lowest of lows, and that responsibility should not be taken lightly.

I'm not here to follow a blueprint or build a business based on what has been done before. I'm here to pave a path. We're pioneers. We lead from the front—trailblazers.

Let's take everything we learned in 2023. The good and the bad. The wins and the losses. Let's learn from all of it as we enter 2024. If you're on this team, you better be here to win because we're not going to try and be the best. We shouldn't be doing it at all. It feels good to win. It feels good to chase down your wildest dreams and aspirations. And it feels even better to do it as a team.

If at any point you are lost, confused, misguided, or unmotivated, I encourage you to raise your hand. Ask for help. We cannot be the best by operating through independent silos. It's time to row the boat in the same direction, with the support of each other, to build the best brand BPN can be.

Be tough. Be really fucking tough.

Go One More.

When I shared that with the BPN organization and the rest of the world, I did not plan, anticipate, or expect what would happen in 2024. So it gives me chills when I think about what happened next. It's another chapter, not just in this book, but in the story of BPN and my entire life.

We kicked off 2023 with the intent to sell a minority share of the business to a private equity partner. I saw it as an opportunity to "de-risk," to take some money off the table by selling a portion of my equity and bringing on a strategic partner that would help us scale the company. After a year-long process, the deal fell apart right before it was planned to be closed and finalized. So, I met with the BPN leadership team, and we had to answer the question "What's next?" Our answer? "We're back to building." No investors? Okay, let's get back to the work without the distractions. Let's redefine our vision, make our values clear, and rebuild the team.

The process put a lot of internal and external stress on the staff. We were trying to ensure we met certain financial metrics that the investors wanted to see, and there were due diligence requests coming in nonstop from the private equity group. That stress trickled down from top to bottom, and everyone could feel the pressure the closer we got to the deal closing.

I had learned more about business in 2023 and 2024 than I had learned in the previous ten years of building BPN. The experience had been extremely rewarding. Yes, it was disappointing to have put in so much work for things to go the way they did. It was frustrating, but I wasn't angry about the deal not happening. I was exposed to a lot of things and learned a lot through the process. I believe that this learning experience happened for a reason. And what a learning experience it was! It felt like being thrown into the deep end of the pool with cinder blocks tied to my ankles and then being asked to stay afloat and swim.

At the start of 2024, I felt a type of passion and energy that I hadn't had since 2019. And 2019 was the year where BPN grew by 400 percent. I had more creative energy, but I had something else: confidence.

I am more capable than I once thought. A lot more capable.

I realized that you don't have to outsource everything. We're all trying to figure it out; no one is any smarter or better than you. Someone might have more experience, but it doesn't mean they are better than you. One of the reasons I stepped down from the CEO role was because I lacked the confidence in my ability to get the business to the next level while simultaneously being the father and husband I wanted to be. I now had the confidence to know I could do both and do them well. Exceptionally well.

Being a pioneer and trailblazer was all I had ever known. The closer we got to completing the deal with the private equity group, the more I realized that this was starting to go against the greatest thing I valued in life: my freedom. The freedom with my time, my energy, where I live, where I work, what I'm working on, and who I'm working with. The private equity deal scared me because it challenged the greatest thing I valued in my life. And no amount of money was worth losing that.

I was reminded how much I love leading people. After stepping down from the CEO role and moving to Nashville, there was a hole inside of me that I could not fill. I tried

everything and anything to fill that hole, yet I could not figure it out. Something was missing. So I started to think back
to the times over the past ten years when I was the most fulfilled. The first thing that came to mind was when I was an
infantry platoon leader leading forty soldiers and noncommissioned officers. I loved serving in the Army, not because
we got to shoot crazy weapon systems or because of all the
training we did, but because I loved leading people. I loved
being a part of a team of selfless individuals who were fighting and serving for a mission, a cause. Being part of a group
that bought into that mission. That's what I loved about the
Army. That's also what I loved about building BPN in the
early days: finding people who wanted to join the team to
fight and win for a cause, a purpose, a mission. That's what
I loved in the beginning. That's what I loved about building
out the team. So when I stepped down from the CEO role, a
part of me died.

I learned that a big part of me needed to lead people.
When those experiences and opportunities were gone, I
missed them significantly. I needed the team, and I needed
to be there with them. So I had a long conversation with my
wife and then spoke to the team, explaining how we needed
to move back to Texas. We had to be close to the business. I
had to put myself in a position to lead the team that I loved
and the business I had spent the last decade building, the
company I had poured my heart and soul into.

If I have learned anything from building a business, it's
that entrepreneurship is all about problem-solving. You're
constantly trying to solve problems. That's what I had been
doing since I first got started, and that was what I had been

doing (or trying to do) in the past year. I had made good decisions and right decisions, but I had also made wrong decisions, ones that didn't result in success or a win. So I knew I had to be decisive, take action, and make decisions, then learn from the outcomes and consequences and pivot. Adapt. Try again. That is what entrepreneurship is all about. That is what life is all about. That is what Go One More is all about.

I had to take ownership of a lot of the things that happened in 2023. At the time, I honestly thought I was making all the right choices, and maybe I was. Maybe they were all the right decisions. Maybe all of the decisions I made and that we made as a team put us in the right place at the right moment for all the right reasons. We'll never know. All I know is how to respond and overcome. To be a problem solver. So I needed to act.

Not only did I know that we as a family and a team had to move back to Texas, but I also knew I had to put myself back in the CEO role. A majority of a leader's job is to teach, develop, and facilitate the growth required for the team. If someone is lost or confused, there's typically a leadership problem at play. And when one person is lost, there are normally a few others to follow. Lost and confused does not lead to rowing the boat in the same direction, and that is inefficient and unproductive.

The entire experience was insightful. It was rewarding. It was challenging. It was emotional. It was all of those things. But I needed that to regain the clarity and focus of what I needed to do next, where the brand needed to move and go, how it needed to adapt and pivot, and how we're going to show up in the future as our true and authentic self.

Chapter Ten

FINISH WELL

"Doubt increases with inaction. Clarity reveals itself in momentum. Growth comes
from progress. For all these reasons, begin."
—Brendon Burchard

At the end of 2023, I invited Lyle Phillips onto my
podcast. Lyle is the pastor of Legacy Church in
Nashville, a church Stef and I attended when we
lived there. During our discussion, I brought up the theme
of one of his recent sermons about finishing a race and asked
him to talk about it more.

"Look, I want to encourage you to finish," Phillips said.
"You may not be able to finish strong, but you can finish well,
and you can finish well by doing good deeds in the process.
Meaning, do things with character. Do things with integrity.
Do things with consistency. Do things with faithfulness to

God, to family, to church. That's how you finish well, even if you don't finish strong. If you've got to crawl over the finish line, crawl, but don't quit."

Those words resonated with me, not just in terms of how you should finish a race, but also how you should pursue your life. When I am on my deathbed, I want to know that I have maintained my character and integrity. I want to rest well knowing I finished well. Sometimes what happens to a lot of people in life is that they get so desperate for the finish line that their values go out the window just to get across it. The people who have always inspired me are those who go through struggles and pain and push through to endure and finish well. Those tough times in our lives are what make us grow and change, as Pastor Phillips explained. He told me, "There's no fruit that grows on the mountaintop. Fruit grows in the valley. The valleys of life are the places of fruitfulness. The places where we stock up. The places where we get fed, the places where we transform. The places where we're changed. I thank God for the valleys. Like, though I walk through the valley of the shadow of death, I will fear no evil. It's the valleys that are the character building."

Now, you may be reading this and think, "Screw that, I'm going to finish strong regardless." And I completely understand and respect that perspective. But sometimes a strong finish isn't going to happen. Sometimes things happen along the way, the plan doesn't go as planned, and your world gets flipped upside down. During those moments, it's easier to quit than to finish. It's easier to give up and give in. Those moments, however, are the ones that define our character. Those are the moments where we get to choose to finish, regardless of the strength we have left. I've watched marathon runners drop out of a race because they weren't on pace for the time they wanted. I've watched entrepreneurs mentally give up on their businesses when their revenue declined and cash got tight. I've seen marriages end in divorce when life got hard and arguments erupted. I've watched people give up on the fight because it got hard. To "finish well" is to reinforce the importance of finishing what you start, regardless of what happens during the process, because the way you do one thing is the way you will do every other thing in your life.

Carve Out the Pain Cave

We usually begin something in hopes of achieving an outcome that is marked by an ending, a finish line. But what if that first step isn't one step closer to the end, but just one part, section, or chapter of our story? As soon as you finish that chapter of your life and turn the page, the next chapter begins. The journey is larger than that one chapter. You must have endurance to make it through the entire story. Each step creates incremental progress toward our greater potential. We finish one thing, not with the goal of ending, but with the intention of creating larger opportunities. As ultramarathon runner Courtney Dauwalter told me once, she is always chiseling out her pain cave and making it bigger. "Every race, I can go in there and make my capacity for that suffering or for pushing through things a little bit bigger by making this pain cave larger in my head."

Our ability to do anything starts with the courage to

begin. We grow by approaching harder challenges with larger goals and greater stakes. It's the process in which we adapt and the momentum we experience that reveals the clarity we need to keep getting stronger and smarter. Go One More is an action, but the true power is from the outcome we experience when that action is amplified with clear and intentional choices.

I started running with the goal of crossing a finish line. As I ran longer and further, that finish line slowly started fading. At some point, it disappeared completely, and what continues to drive me is the momentum created from the opportunities to improve, learn, adapt, and grow.

When I got out of the military in 2017, I said I would never run a day in my life again. That lasted about a year before I felt like a large part of me was missing. I was training hard, and I was training a lot—multiple times a day on some occasions—but the volume wasn't providing me the feeling I was hoping for. Doing more didn't seem to be the solution. I knew I had to "do" differently. Part of my life felt incomplete. I missed the physical struggle I had endured in the Army. I actually contemplated going back in the military for a few months. It felt like my mission wasn't as strong as when I was serving my country, and I wondered if I had made a mistake by leaving the Army. So I started running again. There wasn't a moment where I thought, *You know what? It's running. Running is what I miss. That will fill the holes that I'm experiencing and solve my problems.* No. I just picked up running again. I don't know why. But it changed my life.

As soon as I started running again, I actually started feeling better. At this point in my life, I was in the thick of getting BPN off the ground. We were working nonstop and essentially lived at the warehouse. Stress was at an all-time high as I was trying to manage a scaling business with no outside capital and zero experience or knowledge on how to effectively manage cash flow. There were weeks when our bank account got so low that I didn't know if we would be in business the following month. All of our money was being invested in inventory and tied up with manufacturers or wrapped in pallets or sitting on the shelves of our warehouse. So running found me at the perfect time. It provided me with a moment of silence and solitude from the outside world. It was an escape from distractions, like my phone, email, and meetings. It created the clarity in my mind that allowed me to solve problems we were facing in the organization. Those early runs were critical to positioning my life, BPN, and the growth we experienced where they are today. Running forced me to slow down, think—really think—plan, and attack. When that attack didn't go right, I would think about it on my next run, and then replan and reattack.

I committed to my first marathon in 2018. I've described it as a shit show, a soup sandwich, a mess. It was the Austin Marathon, right in our backyard, a familiar course and an inviting city. I didn't know how to properly train. Honestly, I thought I could just willpower my way through the race. I believed the marathon was more of a mental battle than a physical one; I later realized that if I had trained with a better plan, more volume, and structured workouts, it would have been mentally and physically easier. When I got to mile sixteen, I hit a wall and began to break down. In between walking and jogging, my legs were cramping. I struggled to finish at a time of three hours and fifty-seven minutes. Not the worst time in the world, but I knew I could do better. I knew I didn't prepare in the way I should have, and that bothered me. But despite my poor performance, the energy of that race and the inferior feelings I experienced left a massive impact on me. It was one of the hardest things I had done outside of my Army experiences, and I was humbled.

With the marathon done, I went back to focusing my time on building the business while continuing my consistent strength training. Running wasn't a priority for me. I would run a couple of times a week, maybe a few miles here and there. The following year, as the Austin Marathon approached again, I decided I would give it another attempt. I wanted to revisit that humbling feeling again. I wanted to do something hard. I needed to do something hard. And I wanted to prove to myself that I could do better than the previous year.

Did I change my training? No.

Did I change my mindset? Nope.

Did I really change anything I did the previous year? Uh ... no.

Did I expect to get a better time? Yes.

As you can guess, I ran four hours and fifteen minutes. I actually ran *slower* than the previous year, eighteen minutes slower! The race actually felt more difficult than the 2018 marathon. I knew something had to give.

What am I truly capable of?

What is my full potential?

I wanted to run a faster marathon, but I wasn't committed to making the time that was required in order to actually do it. I said I wanted one thing, but I failed to align my actions with my priorities, and the result I achieved was exactly the one I deserved. I learned that a wish is just a wish as long as you wish for it. So, I made the decision to break that cycle and set a standard for my future self. It was time for a bigger challenge.

"Nick Bare, you are an Ironman."

I wanted to hear that. So that is what I did.

Get to the Finish Line Any Way You Can

I signed up for my first Ironman because of a viral video I saw from the early '80s of an incredible finish of the Ironman in Kona, Hawaii. The video was an example of grit, determination, and will to finish the race, to finish what was started and fight for those last remaining moments. American triathlete Julie Moss entered the 1982 Ironman World Championship not knowing much about the event, so she hadn't sufficiently trained for it. She was leading the event that started with a 2.4-mile swim in the ocean, then continued with 112 miles on bike, and finished with a 26.2-mile run. With less than a mile left to go, her body gave out on her. She crumbled to the ground, then tried to stand but wilted again. The crowd cheered her on, and she was able to get back up and walk, all while looking over her shoulder for her closest competitor.

Ten yards from the finish line, Moss collapsed one final time and had to watch as Kathleen McCartney passed her and finished first. Unable to even stand, Moss literally crawled to the finish line. She did whatever it took to finish the race. That's what made me decide to do the Ironman. I wanted to feel and experience this sort of race. I wanted to be as determined as someone like Moss, who finished despite all her pain and hardship.

So I signed up for Ironman Florida and went all in. I hired a coach. I learned about training and how to build my endurance. I became obsessed with being a student in a space that was so different and new to me. Everything I tried, tested, and learned was shared through the content I created online. And after months of training, I completed my first Ironman in Panama City in November of 2019.

Since then, I've never looked back. I was hooked after seeing the work I was putting in and the results coming out of it. The mental clarity I gained from endurance training gave me a new perspective in everything—my personal life, my professional life, my business, and my relationships. I continued to choose hard things, from triathlons to marathons to ultra-trail races. Each year brings a new opportunity to do something physically challenging that unlocks your greater mental capacity.

In the spring of 2024, the BPN team, myself, and five other runners completed an unsanctioned and unsupported relay race called The Speed Project. This was a race unlike anything else I had done before. A team is made up of four men and two women, and the rules are quite simple: there are no rules. The race started at the Santa Monica Pier in Los Angeles at 4 AM on a Friday, and the goal was for your team to get to Las Vegas as fast as possible. No route, no spectators, no checkpoints, aid stations, or medical tents—nothing. Our team traveled in an RV over the three-hundred-mile journey, while one runner ran at a time. After each runner's two-to-three-mile segment, they would tag out with another runner. It was a crazy experience that took us thirty-five hours and thirty-five minutes.

While the trek was physically challenging and demanding, the race was unique in a much different way. The Speed Project is a massive logistical operation. Each team needs to plan their routes, establish contingency plans, maintain the vehicles, resupply food and water, communicate effectively, build somewhat of a rest schedule, and most importantly, get to Las Vegas safely.

It sounds simple: run from Los Angeles to Las Vegas as fast as possible, but it wasn't. We couldn't run on the freeways or major highways for safety reasons, so our team mapped out a route that we believed we could trust and that was fast. The first hundred miles or so went fast and flawless. The access roads we used were clear, and we were holding a solid pace of six and a half minutes per mile. We were cruising. As you begin to approach the second leg of any ultra, when the sun goes down and nightfall arrives, things change. We went into this race with a plan, but also with the realistic expectation that the plan would probably be thrown out the window at some point. We knew we would have to be adaptable. And adaptable we were.

We were planning to take an off-road trail later on in the race, which would save us forty miles from any of the other routes we could have taken. The plan was to have the RVs push forward at this point and meet us at a rendezvous location. A 4x4 Jeep would take the runners over this off-road segment, which we knew was a well-marked trail from other teams we had talked to who had run The Speed Project in the past. But things changed when we were stopped on our pre-planned route by a "road closed" sign. Our vehicles and runners could not travel on the road that would take us to this off-road trail entrance. So, after studying the map, considering all of our options, and making a new plan, we decided to push off the main road and hop on another off-road trail that would lead us to the original trail we planned to use.

Well, we got lost. The new trail was poorly marked and barely maintained. It was very rocky, rough, and slow-going. Our Jeep was essentially mountain climbing, and I'm not sure how we didn't get it stuck. The runners packed themselves in the off-road vehicles, the drivers were running off zero sleep, and we were losing time. In fact, we were told that our team dropped from fourth place to twenty-eighth place with that detour. It was in this moment that I remembered Pastor Lyle Phillips telling me, "You will not always finish strong, but you can finish well." Although the race at this point felt chaotic and we were losing all the momentum we had created in the previous 150 or so miles, our team still needed to maintain focus and finish well, regardless of whether we lost time, placement, or speed.

We made the decision to pursue a downhill route, which was the rockiest part of the course we had come across yet. We would either get across it to find out what was on the other side or get the vehicles stuck in the middle of nowhere. By the grace of God, the 4x4s made it, and we got back on track. Originally, we had planned to be on the off-road trails for about seven hours, but with the changes to the plan, we had been on the trails for about fourteen hours total. We were exhausted.

After linking up with the RVs, we were able to travel on access roads again and regained speed. For the remaining thirty-eight miles, we switched out runners after every mile and averaged a pace of six minutes per mile all the way into Las Vegas. It was like a marathon training program workout at the end of an ultramarathon. We ended up finishing fourth out of all the other six-person teams.

The message was simple: Finish well.

Vision and Action Produce Momentum

One of my favorite authors, entrepreneurs, and storytellers is Donald Miller. We brought him in to speak with our team about building a brand, clarifying your message, and telling effective stories. It was a highly impactful experience. During his presentation, he talked about the three states of building relationships and how they apply to marketing, but I left thinking about how applicable those three stages are to everything we do in life. The first stage is curiosity, when our interest is sparked by something. The second stage is enlightenment, when we start learning, studying, and educating ourselves on that curiosity. The third state is commitment, when we take action and do something with this curiosity.

Those three stages are necessary in anything we pursue or accomplish. You would never finish a race if you weren't curious if you could do it in the first place. And during that journey of deciding what to do, you would have researched how to successfully complete a race and signed up for one. You would never start a business if you weren't willing to explore a curiosity. If you are reading this book, I'm fairly certain you are in the enlightenment phase of some new chapter or season of life. But each stage needs to be intentional. Each stage requires tremendous thought, time, patience, and clarity in order for the outcomes we want to be as great as possible.

Of all the races I've ever done, the Austin Marathon is my favorite for a lot of reasons. It is the place where I fell in love with running—not just racing but the lifestyle and the activity of running. In 2018, I ran my first marathon, and six years later, in 2024, I was provided the opportunity to deliver the pre-race speech to 19,000 runners at that same marathon. It was an incredible, full-circle moment.

The 2024 Austin Marathon wasn't just a personal full-circle moment. It was full circle for the entire BPN team. Running has transformed my life, and marathons can teach us a lot of lessons about life. The parallels between life and running are so significant that it's hard not to recognize it. Running is hard, and no matter how fast you run or what type of conditioning you have done, marathons are hard, too. They require patience, consistency, and endurance. There are good training days and bad training days. If you go out too hot, you won't be able to sustain the effort and you will break before you cross the finish line. Proper pacing, strategy, intention, and forward thinking are necessary to successfully accomplish a race. And you can keep making progress as long as you keep putting in the work. Nothing is unbelievable, and doubt is only dangerous if you start doubting yourself. Just like Donald Miller explained in his three stages of relationships, you have to be curious about whether you can do it before you commit to seeing for yourself what is possible.

If you would have told me in 2018, as I was lacing up my shoes in preparation to run my first marathon, that I would be delivering the Austin Marathon pre-race speech to 19,000 people a few years later, I would have laughed. I never anticipated or planned for running to become such a big part of my life, but it has. And the only reason I was able to deliver that speech to all of those people was because I had a vision. I consistently amplified that vision with action, and that action produced momentum. It wasn't the end of a story or chapter of my life, but potentially the beginning of a new one.

From the time I ran that first marathon to the time I delivered that pre-race speech, a lot had changed in my life. The business had grown, I met my wife and got married, we had a daughter, I stepped down from the CEO role, and we moved to Nashville. Just a few weeks before that speech, I moved back into the CEO position, our family started preparing to move back to Texas, and my wife was pregnant with our son, Niko. Every action I've taken has been in accordance with a vision that I'm constantly following. Sometimes that vision becomes blurry, and my actions follow suit, but I truly believe that every decision, action, and outcome we experience guides us to become a better version of ourselves, as long as we maintain the self-awareness, perspective, and discipline to learn from our mistakes just as much as our successes.

For a long time, I felt like I made a mistake by stepping down from the CEO role and moving my family out of state, but that decision and those actions ended up creating so much momentum for myself and the team in the long run.

My speech was so much more than a pre-race motivation speech. It was a reflection of my previous year in life and in business, but it was also so applicable to running and especially racing. It was a hard year. But it was meant to be hard. It forced me to grow and become better. At the end of 2023, I was beat up and broke down. Our private equity deal fell apart, I felt lost in my business, and I was ashamed of some decisions I made. And just as my family was finally settling into Nashville after living there for six months, I had to have a hard conversation with Stef about packing up and moving back to Texas. She was also three months pregnant with our second child at this point. It was a wild time. From the outside looking in, many would have said that I finished 2023 strong, but I don't agree. I did, however, finish it well.

The day I delivered that speech was one I will remember for the rest of my life. For me, it was a reminder that this life we live is a process. We will experience highs and lows, successes and failures, wins and losses. We have to endure it all because growth is on the other side. We have to maintain momentum. There was an energy within BPN during this time that I hadn't felt for years. My vision was clearer than ever before, and the actions and decisions I was making were generating momentum.

Another memorable bit of insight Lyle Phillips told me was about the suffering we have to endure when we are training. He shared how his wife followed a runner on social media who was training for a marathon. During one of the runs, this runner's husband, who was riding alongside her, asked if she was hurting. She didn't respond since she was running, but you could see in her face that she was in a lot of pain. So her husband told her, "Your job is to hurt right now. Can you do your job?" I loved that question, so I asked everyone the same thing at the 2024 Austin Marathon. And now, I'm asking you as well. Can you do your job? Can you endure the necessary pain and suffering to get ready for the marathon? For life? To become a better leader, father, mother, husband, wife? A better version of yourself? The best version of yourself?

Sometimes we have to surrender to the pain. That is what causes us to experience growth in our lives. We also need people in our lives who are going to tell us the things we need to hear, even if they are hard to say, people who are going to tell us to "suffer well," as Pastor Phillips explained it.

"I want someone to look me in the eye and say, 'Suffer well, man. Suffer with dignity. Yeah, it's going to suck, but you know what? Do it with dignity. Because that's who you are. And I'm holding you accountable to the greatness that you're called to.'"

Suffer well. Finish well. Do your job.

Go One More Is an Outcome

A significant part of my meaningful mission in life is to share the lessons I've learned from building a business, leading a team, and creating a family. I haven't done it perfectly, and I've made many wrong decisions along the way, but I try to improve and learn from every experience. Those experiences only happen because I embrace growth and the process, and I try to be as intentional as possible with the decisions I make and the mission behind them. Go One More is something I discovered while on a run one day when I was training for a marathon. And those three words not only changed my life, but the lives of many other people, too. They are powerful and have the potential to help you achieve whatever it is that you want. Go One More is much more than an action. It's more than doing one extra rep, working one extra hour, or running one extra mile. All of that extra effort compounds, and it can completely change your life over time, but the effort must be intentional. And we cannot be intentional with our choices when we lack clarity. Go One More is an outcome that we achieve by making highly intentional choices on a consistent basis.

Choose to finish well. Go out there and put in the work and courage required to grow and change your life. Think of it as a marathon, not a sprint. Before you head out to tackle your next goal, I want to leave you with the pre-race speech I gave at the Austin Marathon, the one that brought me back to where this season of my journey began:

"Good morning, Austin, Texas. Later today, people are going to ask you how this race was. And a lot of people are going to respond with, 'It was hard.' The truth is it's supposed to be hard. Races should be hard. We want them to be hard. It forces us to become better. So today, whether you're in the 5K, the half-marathon, or the full marathon, we all have a job to do. That job is to finish the race. Sometimes you're not going to finish strong, but we can finish well. The question is, can you do your job today? Get it done. Full send. Go One More. We'll see you out there."

About the Author

Nick Bare is an entrepreneur, athlete, husband, and father. He founded Bare Performance Nutrition (BPN) out of his college apartment shortly before joining the US Army and serving as an infantry platoon leader. After transitioning out of the military, he continued building BPN, a brand for the committed, to fuel performance and elevate athletic potential. Through his podcast and YouTube channel, Nick has documented his life's journey and lessons learned. The highs and lows, successes and failures, have all been captured and shared through inspiring stories of incredible human achievement. He lives with his family outside of Austin, Texas, and has led his business to become a multimillion-dollar organization.